The Cure

Heal Your Body, Save Your Life

Dr. Timothy Brantley

WILEY

John Wiley & Sons, Inc.

Published by John Wiley & Sons, Inc., Hoboken, New Jersey
Published simultaneously in Canada

Design and production by Navta Associates, Inc.

For general information about our other products and services, please contact our Customer Care Department within the United States at (800) 762-2974, outside the United States at (317) 572-3993 or fax (317) 572-4002.

Wiley also publishes its books in a variety of electronic formats. Some content that appears in print may not be available in electronic books. For more information about Wiley products, visit our web site at www.wiley.com.

Library of Congress Cataloging-in-Publication Data:

Brantley, Timothy.
  The cure : heal your body, save your life / Timothy Brantley.
    p. cm.
  Includes bibliographical references and index.
  ISBN 978-0-471-76825-8 (cloth)
  ISBN 978-0-470-37615-7 (pbk.)
  1. Self-care, Health. 2. Nutritionally induced diseases. 3. Diet in disease.
4. Detoxification (Health) I. Title.
  RA776.95.B735 2007
  613—dc22

                                                            2006016186

Printed in the United States of America

10 9 8 7 6 5 4 3 2 1

I dedicate this book to God, my family and friends,
my godson Cody James Knecht, and all the courageous
people with whom I have worked and from whom
I have learned along this wonderful journey called life.

♡ —a kind person
M.E.C.

CONTENTS

PREFACE

When I was a boy, I sat in a mango tree high above the world, watching squirrels and birds eating directly from nature. I had great love for my family, myself, and all of humanity. Illness was something unexpected that grabbed me by the scruff of the neck and forced me to wake up to a terrible reality. After my mother, my father, and my cousin died tragic deaths at early ages from terminal illnesses, I was motivated to embark on a quest for answers as to why they died so young.

As challenging as it was, I stayed on the path, knowing for sure that God was beside me, guiding me through the bumps in the road and finally leading me to the answers. That same journey drives me forward today, along the path to optimal health, and I want you to know for certain that with the natural bounty available to cleanse and nourish our bodies, no one needs to live in fear of disease.

My research has shown me that most diseases are not mysteries that strike randomly and leave us suffering and bereft with nothing to do and no one to turn to, as we have been falsely conditioned into believing. Rather, I have discovered commonsense answers as to why sickness happens, how to reverse it, and most important, how to prevent ill health in the first place. No matter your background or how your mother or father died, this book will offer you concise answers as to why your loved ones died, why you are sick, and what to do about it, so you don't have to suffer and die like they did.

The sad truth is that the health of North Americans has deteriorated beyond belief in the past hundred years. I often wonder if people fully understand the severity of the health crisis we are all facing. Today, one in every two people develops heart disease and dies from it, while one out of every two and a half people die from some form of cancer. Obesity and diabetes are skyrocketing, most major diseases have increased by leaps and bounds, and the medical and pharmaceutical industries have tried to convince us that poor health and diseases are mysteries. Our kids are succumbing to cancer, diabetes, and even advanced arteriosclerosis, setting the stage for living diseased lives, promising a dismal future for our families and ourselves. And all the while the industrial complex promises to find cures through drugs. My question is, if they never try to find out what causes diseases to take hold and proliferate in the first place, how can they ever find a cure?

While the pharmaceutical companies are busy creating the next synthetic "miracle drug" that they tell us will surely solve the mystery of disease (and reward them financially), I am here to tell you that contrary to popular opinion, there is a logical answer to almost every health condition. Indeed, most illnesses occur as a result of our various bad habits and lifestyles, so no matter how many drugs the industrial complex creates and how many false promises they make, they will never find that miracle drug that will make it go away.

The reason is simple—drugs don't remove the reason they got sick in the first place. Rather, they are like Band-Aids that cover symptoms and placate us, but they can never remove the initial causes of disease. In the meantime, factories pump out more processed foods and drugs that only make us sicker. We need the correct information to take care of ourselves and our children. The state of our health can be turned around with an awareness of what we put in our mouths daily. What we and our families eat will determine whether we remain healthy or suffer prematurely with unnecessary diseases.

Ever since I began my research as a teenager, my clients and friends have been encouraging me to write this book. After all, I've been in the trenches with thousands of sick and dying patients, researching and helping them find the underlying factors that created their health challenges in the first place. I knew that I would offer my findings to the public at some point, but up to now I wasn't ready, sure that I was missing some of the pieces. Now, after two decades of dealing with terminal illness with my clients, I am ready to offer you my life's work, the culmination of my experience in working with the sick and the dying.

As I share my simple, profound truths with you that will allow you to restore balance and vitality to your system, please follow the keys and the road map back to optimal health. It is my sincere wish that the answers within might start a grassroots movement to educate the masses.

Imagine the beauty of a world in which every man, woman, and child understands the simplicity and the profundity of living in accordance with nature!

Eating Creation's healing foods from the land and the sea has always been my passion. Now it's time we all got back to our roots in the soil as we consume our perfect food and drink as Creation made it, unspoiled by human manipulation.

Please understand that this book has been written not as a complicated guide that only doctors and health professionals can understand, but rather for you. My goal is for you to understand why and how you got in trouble with your health in the first place and what to do about it, because believe it or not—you already have the key that can unlock the door to great health! The choices you make today will determine whether you and your children will be sick in the future or will enjoy the optimal health our Creator had in mind for us.

You will find a variety of stunning true case studies woven throughout the text of this highly informative book, in which my clients successfully turned around some of the most devastating health conditions by cleansing their bodies and being nourished by God's foods. Whether you are reading this book as a learning tool, as an inspiration, or as both, please take heart. Help is on the way, and even if you are facing the most serious cases of imbalance and illness, this book will show you how to turn around disorders naturally.

My life has been one big treasure hunt where one clue led to another, to another, and then another, with God beckoning just ahead of me, waiting for me to catch up. And somehow, one step at a time, after all these years, I think I'm finally doing it. In this book I'm sharing with you for the first time the answers that God and my research have given me. If you follow His road map and listen to your body, you will find my systems and formulas to be the perfect and indisputable lifesavers they have been for me and so many others searching for our birthrights of optimal health—both on the inside and out.

ACKNOWLEDGMENTS

This was not an individual effort. It was a team effort.

I would first and foremost like to thank Kristin Rotblatt for working day and night, helping me write this book. Without her amazing writing, editing, and communication skills, I really do not know how I would have accomplished this. Her talents never cease to amaze me, and her contributions are never-ending. Kristin is an acupuncturist by profession and has studied nutrition for the past twenty-five years. I was the beneficiary when she came to me as a client looking for help with her health. Kristin has been the most dedicated and loyal friend anyone could dream of having in a lifetime. She is truly a gift, and I have the deepest admiration for her in all respects. She is not only one of the kindest, most loving, and most thoughtful people I have ever known, she is also one of the most talented. If anyone is fortunate enough to have a friend like this in their lifetime, they will have had a successful life. Kristin's abilities and talents continue to boggle my mind. The way she challenged my thought processes, captured the information, and helped me transfer the words to paper was magical. On top of that, her editing skills stunned me.

I also want to thank Kristin's husband, Steven Rotblatt, their daughter, Corey, and their son, Max for being so patient and understanding when she spent so much of her family time helping me get this message out.

Sincere thanks to Andrea Cagan, master writer, for her expertise, loving support, and encouragement. She was an essential part of the writing team and definitely added her special magic to the writing of this book. Without her immense skills and experience, this process would have been overwhelming. Her faith in me spurred me forward, and her excitement about my work was very much appreciated.

I wish to thank Thomas W. Miller, executive editor of general interest books at John Wiley & Sons. Tom understood me immediately and got what I was about. He shared and supported my vision of wanting to educate and enlighten the public about the body's inherent ability to heal and cure itself. His feedback was brilliant, and he was like a great guidance counselor. Also a thank you to Juliet Grames, Tom's assistant.

Thanks to my agent, Richard Abate at ICM, and Kate Lee, his associate, who always look out for my best interests.

I want to thank Sylvester Stallone, who has been a great supporter and champion of mine. He was willing to step up and open the door for me.

Thanks to Steve Knecht for his loving support, his loyal friendship, and his expertise in everything. He is a huge rock in my life, and his brilliance in business has inspired me over the years. His entire family has shown me so much love, "adopting" me as one of their own.

I want to thank Christine Storey for her wonderful support and friendship.

I wish to thank my brother, Douglas Brantley, for loving me and always being there with his encouragement and support.

I want to thank my uncle, Bob Brantley, for his unconditional love and support from the time I was a little boy. His tireless search for truth was instrumental in setting the course of my life. His generosity and the example he set as he selflessly gave to countless others will always be an inspiration.

Finally, I owe a debt of gratitude to all my clients who led me down this amazing path of discovery. Their cases helped to piece together the puzzle of my life's work. I also want to thank all the men and women who have been my teachers. Their courage, passion, and commitment to truth have encouraged and guided me every step of the way.

PART ONE

The Search for Balance

CHAPTER 1

Balance and Imbalance

I was fortunate to be raised in Miami, Florida, in the midst of a very large park. Grassy hills behind our house cascaded down into the park grounds, where I inhaled the scent of freshly mowed grass. Our grounds were filled with enormous trees that I climbed every chance I got, including a coconut tree in our front yard, and grapefruit, key lime, and mango trees in the back. There I would sit on the tallest branches with the squirrels and birds who were squawking and fighting each other for the ripening fruit. My own private Eden.

What a place to grow up and escape from the rest of the world! There, from high above, I could almost see the distant whitecaps on the turquoise ocean waves, and I inhaled the salty, fresh air and the aroma of maturing fruit. I felt connected to the earth back then, watching things grow and ripen like I was an explorer making new discoveries every day.

I also felt calm and serene when I worked with my dad in our garden, watching plump vegetables grow from a tiny seed without any help from us besides water and love. Nature seemed to have all the answers. It had been harmonious, balanced, and filled with vitality since the beginning . . . whenever that was.

My dad, Cecil, who was raised on a farm in Georgia, taught me all about the beauty and balance of nature. Extremely poor, his family had lived off what they could grow. The soil was everything to them, and judging from how great my dad looked and how strong he turned out, it was more than enough. No killing himself lifting weights to achieve a buff look for my dad! Genetics were good to Cecil Brantley, and he was quite a physical specimen, with luminous green eyes, pitch-black wavy hair, a strong, healthy body, and a powerful chest.

My older brother, Douglas, also was in love with the earth. Although we were like night and day (he was quiet and laid-back while I never stood still), we tilled the soil together with my dad. Our vegetable garden was an example of how my dad taught us to respect nature. I'd make a little mound of earth, put in that tiny seed, and when it would sprout, I'd be amazed, making my family laugh each time I cried out, "Oh, my God, the little green thing is coming out."

Dad made sure that Douglas and I worked with him, weeding, digging, preparing the land for planting and finally watering. "This is where it all comes from, boys," he'd say as we toiled and sweated in the garden. "God has all the answers, so just keep digging."

My dad didn't entirely live an idyllic life, however. He had escaped a tough childhood by going to war. When his tour of duty was over, he returned home to become a firefighter and the owner of his own small exterminating company. Many a morning he returned from a twenty-four-hour shift smelling like a wave of ashes. When it had been a really big fire, his eyes were red and you could pick up the scent of burning hair on his head, arms, and eyelashes. If he looked visibly shaken, I knew someone had died in the fire, but he never talked about it. He just drank his sorrows away.

In complete opposition to the garden of Eden just outside our home was our kitchen pantry. It was was something else altogether. At the time, none of us thought it was strange that the fresh produce from our garden, nature's undisputed miracles, were hidden beneath an overwhelming amount of packaged, dead, refined, overprocessed foods. We and almost everyone else ate the Standard American Diet, which has come to be called SAD for reasons that I would understand much later.

Television commercials and advertising campaigns influenced my parents, as they did most people in the country, creating a war zone in our kitchen. Alongside the freshest fruit in the world, the shelves and countertops were littered with junk and processed foods, such as boxes of sugared refined cereals, white bread (lots of it), white crackers, hydrogenated oils such as vegetable shortening, pasteurized milk, and all kinds of canned goods poisoned with deadly preservatives. And then there were the desserts—white sugary pastries, glazed donuts, candy bars of all sorts, ice cream, Popsicles, and sodas galore.

The irony was that amid all the sugar, artificial sweeteners in pink and blue packaging, refined salt, additives, and food coloring that took up space in our kitchen cabinets, my mother banned packaged, powdered instant drinks that came in strange colors. "They're not healthy for you," said my mom, biting into a piece of white toast with margarine, powdered artificial sweetener, and jelly.

My mother, Violet, was from a poor background like my father's. She was a product of a large family who always struggled to keep food on the table. As a result, my brother and I were expected to eat whatever our parents fed us. It was not an option to reject any kind of food; you simply ate it, and you'd better be thankful. I believed in gratitude as my parents did—I still do—but back then, processed and refined foods were the mainstay diet in most American households, and our house was no different.

I ate what I was told. Why shouldn't I? I felt good, I had tons of energy, and I spent as much time outdoors as possible, fishing, diving, and bouncing through the ocean waves, the salt water hitting my face as I breathed in the fresh air. Nature was all around me, and I played hard, ate as much as I wanted, stayed slim, and was the picture of health—or so I thought. Even though there was always more than enough food to fill my belly, in truth I was undernourished, literally starving, and nobody knew it—until my body began to rebel.

As a kid, I rarely got sick besides the normal childhood illnesses such as measles, mumps, and chicken pox. I got over them like all the other kids did, and I almost never missed school, although I was hit with unexplained physical symptoms, such as waking up with a stuffy nose, occasional constipation, and an embarrassing skin condition that caused me great physical pain.

I was seven when I noticed white, dry scales on my feet that kept getting bigger. They cracked and bled, looking reptilian enough for me to never take off my shoes in public. The worst part was how much they hurt. My feet were always in radical pain, and at times I could barely walk. This prompted a visit to the doctor; my parents assured me, "Don't worry, the experts will handle this."

Apparently his white coat made my pediatrician an expert, and I was willing to go along with him if he could help me. He declared my foot problem to be a fungus and gave me some cream to rub on it. Then I did the unthinkable.

"What caused it?" I asked, to the horror of my parents. My mother reached over and put her hand over my mouth. I hated that, but I was used to it. She did it to me whenever I asked a so-called authority the question. Why? She considered it a sin to question the experts, and every time I did so, she was devastated.

The white-coated god ignored my impertinent question, so I took the cream and left with my mother. Two weeks later, however, when the cream didn't work and my feet got worse, it was back to another doctor, this time a big, fat man with glasses who also was wearing the white coat. He took a thorough look at my scaly feet and said, "You have a fungus."

I'd already heard that from the last guy.

He went on, "Here's some cream that should control it, but you'd better get used to it because you'll probably have it for a long time."

Then I did it. "What caused it?" I asked.

"I never thought about that," he said, smiling.

"Why not?" I asked.

With that, my mother shot me a look and put her hand over my mouth again. The minute we left the doctor's office that day, my mother smacked me on the head for questioning the doctor. I'd been dubbed "Why Timothy" from the moment I could talk, and even though adults generally answered, "Because I told you so," I didn't stop asking questions.

You can probably guess what happened next. The second medication didn't work either. And for a ten-year-old, it was tough. My skin condition continued to get worse over the next three years. More visits to "experts" (this time they were called specialists) did nothing for me. Each "specialist" sounded like a machine that had been built and programmed in the white-coat factory. They usually ended up handing me a cream, often the same one the last doctor had prescribed, and sent me home.

When it got really bad, a doctor recommended that I sleep with plastic bags wrapped around my feet to make sure the medicine was soaking all the way in. I wondered why I should bother, since the medication clearly was not working, but I gave it my best try, all the while wondering if maybe the experts were having a bigger problem than I was. They didn't seem to know what to do for me, and they wouldn't admit it, but I knew if I voiced my doubts, my mom would kill me. Instead, I hid my feet from everyone, and eventually my parents refused to spend any more money taking me to doctors. My condition, they figured, was not life threatening and I needed to learn to live with it.

Surgery

When I was thirteen, I was still careful never to remove my shoes and socks in public. Then my headaches started. They were persistent, and I wondered if they had something to do with my dad's exterminating business. Doug and I helped him and we kidded around, accusing him of using us as cheap labor. We were around some of the most toxic chemicals known to man, such as malathion, Dursban, chlordane, and DDT before it was outlawed. These kinds of pesticides lay around our garage in unsealed barrels, and we used the stuff to spray lawns and kill fleas, roaches, and any other unfortunate bugs that happened to be living in the vicinity. I squeezed through dark crawl spaces under people's homes to kill termites, sometimes rubbing against house boards as a spiderweb full of dead bugs fell into my hair. In case the bogeyman showed up, I was ready with my spray gun to blast him full of poison!

Doug and I were often under houses for hours, digging trenches against the walls and pumping gallons of chlordane in there. When we crawled back out again, wet from the poison and sweat, our faces were swollen and our eyes were red and burning. Pumpkin Head, we'd call each other as my dad washed us off with the hose.

"It's just a little poison, boys," he said, laughing. "It isn't gonna kill you."

My headaches got worse, but my parents didn't know what else to do. Whatever happened or however we felt, we all went to church on Sunday, unless my dad was fighting a fire somewhere. I respected the fact that he and my mom spent time helping the poor and the needy through our church, but as my mother felt the need to continuously impose her will on her family and her husband, the relationship between my parents became strained.

When my father drank, I escaped to the park outside our house, where I scurried up the tallest tree and lost myself in nature. I felt better, but nothing helped my headaches, which intensified as time passed. So did the huge scales on my feet, but my problems were soon over-shadowed when my mother found a lump in her breast. For many months, the lump never changed in size. She wanted to forget about it, but her friends pressured her until she went to see an expert for a diag-nosis. He took a biopsy and soon informed my mother that although the lump was small and had not grown for months, she had breast cancer. Her worst fears were realized. Her visit to a second specialist confirmed the diagnosis, and both doctors agreed that she needed to have a radical mastectomy.

"They know what to do," my mother assured me, looking more ter-rified than I'd ever seen her. "Whatever the doctor says goes."

"But why do they want to cut off your breast?" I asked, angering my mother with one more "why" question.

Her answer was predictable. "Because they're the experts and they know what to do."

When my mother came out of surgery after one of her large breasts had been removed, she looked deformed. Her chest was concave on one side, and she was in so much pain, they kept her drugged out of her mind. She was never the same after that. Instead of the strong, willful, energetic taskmaster, she was more like a bird with a broken wing and spirit, despite the fact that the god in the white coat soon declared her healed.

"It was a success," the doctor told us. "We got all the cancer, and the margins are clear."

"What does that mean?" I asked. Even in my mother's drugged-out state, she managed to shoot me a look.

The doctor explained that they had cut out the surrounding tissue where cancer cells could be hiding. "We didn't find any," he said with a smile on his face.

"Doctor," I said, "why did she get cancer to begin with?"

My mother apologized to him as he said to me, "Well, son, we don't know why."

"Don't you want to know?" I said. I was already in trouble.

"I think that's enough questions, young man," he said with irritation in his voice.

My mom glared at me. Once again, I had committed an unpardonable sin in my family, punishable by the belt. I'd questioned authority, and it was a bad night for me when we got back home. I was soundly beaten by my dad as they continued to throw the word "remission" around. They said it meant that the cancer had stopped growing. So why didn't they look happy? At my mom's next appointment, remission or not, the doctor prescribed radiation treatments "to discourage the cancer from coming back."

"But if she's in remission," I said, "why are you giving her radiation?"

My mother and the doctor looked like they wanted to wring my neck, but I didn't care. This made no sense to me. I couldn't fit the pieces of the puzzle together, they didn't fit, and I would never stop trying.

I was told that radiation was a process by which they fried cells, the cancer cells *and* the good ones, to prevent the cancer from ever returning. Once again, I was filled with questions. If this process was safe and effective for someone who was in remission, then why didn't they give radiation to everyone, just to make sure cancer never attacked them? Why didn't the doctors, their wives, and their children take radiation as a preventive measure? I pictured a radiation drive-thru like a fast-food window.

They literally fried my mother's chest with what I would later discover was an enormous amount of radiation therapy. When I saw the radiation burns on my mother's chest, I wondered if no treatment at all would have been a better bet. I heard her crying from pain in the night, and I asked God to send it to me instead of her. When they declared her treatments over, I sighed with relief, but the damage was done. She spent the next year trying to recover, but although the pain lessened, she was devastated at how her body looked. Friends pretended everything was normal, but we all knew better. The cancer was back!

Once again, my escalating foot condition and headaches took a backseat to the fact that my mother began to undergo chemotherapy. "If you don't do chemo," they warned her, "the cancer will spread all over your body."

And if you do the chemo? I wanted to ask but didn't. I also didn't say, "Look what these treatments are doing to her." No one said that and no one would, except my brother and I, and no one listened to us anyway.

As my mother jumped from the frying pan of radiation into the fire of chemotherapy, she became sicker than I'd ever seen her. Her hair fell out, her arms swelled beyond recognition, and the nausea and dizziness were constant. She hardly slept, and she cried, moaned, and vomited all night long. Doug was away at university, and the bogeyman whom I previously had feared when the house was dark and quiet seemed like a good alternative to the agony I heard coming from my mother. I prayed for the dark and the quiet, even for the bogeyman to distract me, but my sleep was interrupted every night for months by the sounds of my mother's illness and treatments. How she survived the chemo, even for a little while, is still a mystery to me. Her genetics must have been such that she was able to get through the worst treatments in the world, which they all thought were keeping her alive. I wasn't so sure.

Everyone was talking about remission again, but if this was the same as the remission from the radiation, I didn't believe she was okay. At this time, a health professional whom I liked, an elderly nutritionist in his seventies named Dr. Jackson, came to the house to give my mother vitamin B_{12} shots. She got a temporary lift from them, and I wanted to bombard him with questions. I believe he would have answered them, but I never had an opportunity to be alone with him.

While my brother and I joked about Mom's wig that reminded us of coconut hair they used on mannequins in department stores, we looked around us to find some disturbing answers. We knew a few adults who had gone through the same treatments, and they were dying. My common sense and instincts were telling me one thing, while all of their doctors were saying something else. When I realized that nature was in balance but the doctors were not, I thought about my cousin Debbie.

As a teenager, she'd gotten cancer, which inspired the doctors to put her on not one or two but five different types of chemotherapy. Her dad, my Uncle Bob, was beside himself with anger when he discovered that one of the drugs had actually caused new tumors to grow. The treatments *were* killing her, just as Doug and I had suspected. We tried to talk some sense into my dad, using Debbie as an example, but he only got more confused. He would not believe us when we told him that chemotherapy could actually cause cancer to grow.

As my cousin Debbie's health continued to decline, Uncle Bob decided to take matters into his own hands. He advised my father to take my mother off all traditional treatments, and he took his daughter to a clinic in Mexico run by a medical doctor called Dr. Contreras. Unfortunately, the doctor told Uncle Bob that Debbie's immune system was too compromised after so much chemo to respond to alternative treatments. But Uncle Bob kept looking, even when conventional doctors declared the physicians at alternative clinics to be frauds and quacks.

When I asked him why these natural-therapy doctors were in Mexico, he explained that they had no choice. They were persecuted, prosecuted, and imprisoned in the United States for treating people with unorthodox therapies that were actually helping them. Then Uncle Bob told me about laetrile, which he believed was healing some people with cancer.

"It's derived from apricot pits," he said, "and people are getting results." He told me that it was illegal in the United States because it threatened big business.

I'd suspected as much, but when I heard the unadulterated truth from my Uncle Bob, an undeniable truth-teller, the reality was hard to swallow. Big business was making money off cancer patients, blocking all competition, and refusing to accept any therapies that did not pump up the bank accounts of the pharmaceutical industry executives.

Next, we heard about a man named Dr. Burton, an American doctor who had devised a plan to help rebuild the blood of people with cancer, and who had been shut down by the medical authorities. His work focused on replacing nutrients that were missing from an ill person's bloodstream. He had some success, but he moved to Jamaica, where he was allowed to practice. I couldn't understand why the medical establishment refused to acknowledge his work, but they wanted him gone. It was a huge red flag for me. I was swiftly learning that the medical industry, often corrupt and closedminded, was not usually interested in curing people. Rather, it seemed to me that they were interested in profiting from disease, stopping any practitioner who had a possible answer. My eyes were opening, and I hated what I was seeing.

It was too late for my cousin Debbie, since her immune system was shot to hell, but would an alternative treatment work for my mother? We found a biochemist named Dr. Carey Reams, who did pH tests (acid vs. alkaline) of a person's saliva and urine. His theory was that if a person's pH balance was kept within or brought back to an optimal range, that person would become disease-free. We tried to contact him, but to no avail. Like Dr. Burton, he was under constant scrutiny by the medical authorities as they hassled, persecuted, and eventually prosecuted him for practicing medicine without a license. In other words, if the therapies worked, the doctor was doing something illegal, especially if he used no drugs at all, only herbs, vitamins, minerals, and dietary changes. When Dr. Reams refused to stop helping people, he was tossed in prison over and over again. What kind of power did the medical authorities have to manipulate the system like that and put in jail doctors who had a clue how to offer help and relief to sick people with no hope?!

I was stunned. This was America, supposedly the land of the free. Where was our freedom to choose treatments when we got cancer or any other disease? It was all a myth. We were not free to heal ourselves as we saw fit, or to use anything that nature had created to feel better. It seemed like we had no health care system at all. When I fully understood that our government was more interested in working with the industries to make money than it was in healing people, I succumbed to the anger, disappointment, and awareness that were flooding me. I refused to go along with it. I was heading out to sea, my course set to discover a brand-new world where things made sense and people treated each other with the profound respect that nature and each and every one of us needs and deserves.

I was surprised at my mother's devastation when the cancer came back a third time. What did she expect after exposing her insides to some of the most toxic chemicals on earth? I barely blinked when I heard them telling her she had to undergo yet another round. I was accustomed to the doctor's MO by now and I was swiftly losing faith in the system.

"But I got so sick from the last round, I got worse," my mother said.

"Well," said the doctor, "I know it seems that way, but we have to get this cancer back under control."

As if they ever had her cancer in control in the first place! My mother sat there, wide-eyed like a mouse stuck in a trap, nodding her head in agreement. I looked straight ahead. Did the doctors think we were all idiots, as mindless as sheep walking off a cliff because the leader did it? All of a sudden, "Why Timothy" reared his head as I asked, "What about trying some natural forms of treatments like herbal formulas?" My mother's gaze pierced through me.

The doctor retorted, "Don't listen to those quacks and frauds. That stuff could kill her."

It became clear to me in that moment that most doctors had lost their ability to think creatively a long time ago. They were programmed and conditioned by the pharmaceutical industry, and they resented my questions because they didn't know the answers. Uncle Bob was right. It was all about the money. They were not interested in competitive and alternative methods of healing and watching people get well because there was no financial gain involved.

When I turned my attention back to the doctor, I thought *he* was the quack, not the rest of the world, and I laughed out loud.

"Something wrong here, son?" he asked, clearly annoyed that I was amused by something in such a serious moment.

Everything was wrong, but like a respectful, well-trained son, I said, "No, sir."

"Good," he said brusquely, "that'll be all for today." He got up and walked out of the room. The odd thing was that I suddenly felt excited. If the doctors were so terrified of nondrug therapies, they must work! I left the office determined to find out everything I could about the "quacks and frauds" of the world—the real healers. But first I needed to talk some sense into my dad.

"Dad," I said, "first Mom got butchered and then she got fried and poisoned. I'm sick of the doctors' stupid words: chemotherapy, radiation, remission. None of it is working. Can't you see they're killing her faster than the cancer ever could? How stupid do they think we are?"

My dad looked like he wanted to rip my head off, and I felt the hair on the back of my head stand on end. We locked eyes for what seemed like an eternity—until his expression suddenly changed. He dropped his gaze to the ground. "They're doing the best they can," he told me in a weak voice. "It just isn't working."

I sat on the couch beside my dad. "They're not doing their best," I said. "They always claim that the health of the patient is the most important thing, right? Then why are they threatened by other treatments that might work? Look what happened to Debbie as soon as she started chemo. No one can help her now. Look at what happened since Mom got radiation and chemo. She keeps getting worse. Enough is enough!" I said.

He shook his head, got up, and walked out of the room.

.   .   .

The next round of chemo made my mother so sick, she threw up profusely, her throat was swollen all the time, and she moaned all night long. I thought my lack of sleep at night was causing my inability to stay awake in school, something that plagued me the most right after lunch. I still wonder why it never occurred to me that my eating habits might be causing my desire to fall asleep. Today they would probably call the problem attention deficit disorder (ADD) and prescribe a drug. Back then, I lived with it, struggling to stay awake until the sugar in my system was finally under control.

The doctors pumped my mom full of a drug mixture they called Bromptins' Mix. It was predominantly morphine and she felt so little after she took it, she would doze off and sleep. In her waking state, she fell in and out of coherence. She'd start talking about something and suddenly say, "I was hallucinating. Sorry."

Just when I thought it couldn't get worse, my dying mother had become an incoherent morphine junkie. When I heard that Dr. Jackson was coming back to give my mother a vitamin B_{12} shot, I couldn't wait to see the look of horror on his face when he saw what the doctors had done to her. I met him outside where I could talk to him alone and prepare him for what he was about to see.

"They're killing her," I told him.

"I've seen this quite a bit," he said calmly.

"My uncle is trying to get some laetrile," I said. "Maybe we could inject her."

"It's too late," Dr. Jackson told me. "Her veins are in such bad shape from the chemo, even if you smuggled it in and we tried it, her veins are so collapsed, it would be really hard to inject it. Besides, I can't administer it because it's illegal. I'd lose my license."

I stared at him, unable to respond as my mom slowly hobbled out the front door and stood to face us. "Hi, Dr. Jackson," she said. "I'm walking. This must be my lucky day."

Dr. Jackson looked at me and said, "Keep up the good work, Timothy. You have great instincts." And he helped my mother back to bed.

Over the following weeks, I watched the life draining out of my mother as her body was being poisoned and depleted. When she tried to vomit and nothing came out, she described the feeling as having her intestines ripped out. To me, it looked like a python was slowly tightening its grip on my mother's neck, squeezing the breath out of her.

I lost myself in glazed jelly doughnuts, chocolate milk, sodas, and pizza. I was obsessed with understanding what had caused the cancer, and I began to delve more deeply into the suggested diets from alternative therapists. They all had three things in common: naturalness, simplicity, and safety, a far cry from the toxic drugs and chemical therapies the doctors were prescribing.

At this point, the simple act of walking hurt and my headaches were becoming intolerable, and I decided to take a big step and see a doctor on my own, since all our family money was being used to keep my mother alive.

I was a teenager when I made the appointment with the doctor who had been my pediatrician since I was a kid. I hoped he could help. "It's my feet, "I said. "They're worse than before, and I have some wicked headaches to go along with them." I showed him my scales.

"Wow!" he said. "No foot modeling this week. You could scare away the buzzards."

We both laughed until he said, "Let's try this other cream. It's stronger than the last one, so if your feet don't fall off, it might work."

"And if it doesn't?" I asked.

"I have a saw at home," he teased. "If all else fails, we can cut them off."

I appreciated his sense of humor, since I hadn't laughed in a long time. He was so jovial, I took a chance and said, "I've been looking into diets and nutrition lately and I wonder if it has some connection to my problem. Also, what about the pesticides? I was exposed to a lot when I was a kid. What do you think?"

I was encouraged when, unlike other doctors I'd seen, he acted unthreatened by what I was saying to him. He even seemed to be thinking about it. "Well," he said, "the pesticides may have irritated your feet somewhat back then, but not now. Why don't you try some different brands of aspirin for the headaches and see what works best?"

"I was thinking," I tried to explain, "about the kinds of foods I've been eating. Isn't it possible that my diet could be causing it? Maybe Mom's diet is bad for her, too."

"No," he said, smiling, "I'm afraid that's not it. Try the cream and if your feet fall off, don't call me."

I left the office laughing and frustrated at the same time. If the gentlest, kindest doctor of all had written me off, it was obvious they were all too programmed and conditioned. The doctor I'd just seen had been taught to prescribe drugs endorsed by the U.S. Food & Drug Administration and nothing else. When I applied the doctor's stronger cream, it calmed some of the itching but did nothing to stop the cracking.

As my headaches intensified, so did the stress at home. My mother now required oxygen to breathe, and her lungs were filling with fluid. The sound of her lungs crackling as she tried to suck in air through the oxygen mask echoed throughout our small house. It was back and forth to the hospital as her arms and legs wasted away. To this day, I'm haunted by the image of her holding her wig in place as I carried her into the bathroom. I remember thinking how mangled and sideways our lives had become, just like her wig.

My studies about food and natural healing taught me that not only should processed foods be excluded from a sick person's diet, but also that no human being should be eating them. Most medical doctors considered eating whole foods to be a radical approach, constantly reminding me about quacks and frauds, but this was my final shakedown. At this point I knew my mother was a lost cause, since her immune system was virtually gone, but I needed the information for myself.

I got teased to no end, both in school and at home, when I started passing on foods that contained sugar and white flour. It was never easy for me. It was tough, like a junkie trying to get off heroin. I craved sugar, and when I ate vegetables instead, my dad and my friends suggested I go outside and graze on the front lawn. Neither of my parents, even my mom in her present condition, could fathom why I was changing my diet. I told them over and over but they were too stuck in their ways to understand that I was looking for relief, plain and simple.

When I observed my friends' and family's reactions to my new, healthier diet, I realized how thoroughly we'd been programmed by the food industry. It made no difference to them that I was getting clearer while my mother was becoming a zombie, too incoherent from the drugs to talk to me at all. The doctors were giving her drugs to cope with other drugs, as our medical bills escalated while my mother's health plummeted.

One evening at the hospital, she looked at me through her big brown eyes and squeezed my hand. Then she passed out. I stared at the tubes hanging from her arms covered with bruises, the oxygen mask covering her face. If this was survival, I wanted no part of it. We as a society had gone off the deep end, allowing ourselves to be controlled by an industry that didn't seem to care about how their treatments were affecting our overall health.

I left my mother in the hospital that night, with thoughts swirling through my head. The house was quiet, I fell asleep almost immediately, and I was in the midst of a profound dream when a warm wave rolled over my body. My eyelids opened slowly, as if by themselves, and I felt a deep sense of calm and serenity. I lay there quietly, watching the sun rise, waiting for the phone to ring. When it did, my dad picked it up, said a few words of thanks to someone, and walked into my room. His voice choked. He gathered himself for a second and managed to say, "Your mother just passed away."

I looked out the window at the sky. "I know," I said.

It was unbearable to look at my father's face, his pain mixed with relief that the agony was over. I felt as if a giant spear had passed through my body and left a gaping hole as I got out of bed. I staggered outside to the front lawn and lay there on my back. "Thank you, God," I said, "for taking my mother out of her pain and suffering."

I cried into the grass, grateful that her ordeal was over. She was free and so was I, to continue my quest to learn the truth about healing, a cause to which I would dedicate my life.

CHAPTER 2

My Quest for Truth

I lay there on the lawn for some time, feeling the sun warm my grief-stricken body. Years of stress, lost sleep, struggle, suffering, and frustration at not being heard, bubbled to the surface. I stared up at the sky. It was over now, my mother was at peace, but there was no rest for me, it seemed, as I rose to my feet and walked back into the empty house.

The ever-present whir of the oxygen tank was gone, there was no more yelling, whispering, begging, pleading, and panicking, since death had finally claimed my mother. I wandered from room to room, as if to reacquaint myself with my new surroundings. The serenity for which I'd prayed should have been there, but I didn't feel free, peaceful, or serene.

I recalled one day, close to the end, when I'd knelt down in front of my mother, trying to assist Dr. Jackson in finding a vein in her arm that had not collapsed from chemotherapy. As each unsuccessful prick of her arm made her flesh turn purple and bleed, I knew there was no hope for her survival. My mom looked so open and gentle, the tears running down her face, I didn't want her to see that I was losing faith, but I didn't know how to hide it. My mom looked over at me and said quietly, "Are you okay, Bud?" I pretended I was fine.

"Please," she said. "You have to do everything you can to stop this disease. Find a way. Use that lightbulb of a mind that God gave you, because no one deserves to suffer like this."

Those were some of her last words to me, and after she was gone, I heard them every time I went to sleep, got up, took a shower, went to work, or did anything else. I was haunted, left with all of my unanswered questions piled on top of the grief of watching my mother suffer and finally losing her.

This was a pivotal moment in my life when I strengthened my commitment to my mother and myself to keep searching for answers to these "mysterious" diseases. I had found my passion that would set the course of my life and I knew that the answers to my questions did not lie in conventional medicine, where all the doctors ever did was run tests, prescribe drugs, and perform surgery. What about healing people? What about discovering causes? What about changing our basic overall physical conditions to fight degenerative diseases?

My father looked fragile after so much hardship and tragedy, and I feared for his health as he struggled with a mountain of medical bills that kept him awake at night, worrying. I'd already lost my mother, and the idea of losing him next, the man whom I dearly loved and respected, motivated my search for truth.

I embraced it as a giant jigsaw puzzle. I needed to find one piece at a time until one day I would fit it all together into a logical whole that made sense. I would never again view the pharmaceutical community in the same light, although I did see areas where traditional medicine, as it was, could be helpful. I recognized the merits of this system when it came to crises or traumas such as accidents, emergency surgeries, orthopedics, lacerations, gunshot wounds, broken bones, and similar things. I could even understand the wisdom of drugging the body temporarily to alleviate excruciating pain. Conventional treatment for these kinds of acute problems was valid in my estimation. I knew there were some strengths in most systems, and I didn't want to throw out what was good along with what wasn't.

On the other hand, my mother's agonizing and extended death opened my eyes to how much the system, in its irresponsibility and motivation for money, could do harm rather than heal. It seemed to me that the worst part was that the people touting the system did very little to search out and remove causes for diseases. To take it one step farther,

I saw that they not only avoided looking at causes, they also refused to admit that their system was failing their patients.

My father was forced back into the exterminating business to pay the daunting bills that had mounted during my mother's long illness, and I joined him to help out. Now I continued to poison myself with chemicals while I searched for a way to detoxify my body. But what else could I do? My dad was my only parent now, and I worked by his side in the blistering Miami heat and intense humidity with chemicals that could take your skin off, because I feared he'd drop dead of a heart attack. My dad may have been strong in the past, but life had taken its toll, and the unrelenting financial stress was buckling his body and his spirit.

When I visited my neighbors after my mother's death, I discovered that most people had no idea what was going on when it came to their health. Here we all were, proud to be living in a so-called free and democratic society, but really, where did freedom go when someone became ill? What had happened to the doctor's Hippocratic oath "to do no harm"?

What was the first piece of the puzzle that would form a healing foundation for what was to come? Once again, I pushed my own health problems into the background, focusing on helping my father while I kept my vow to my mother to find answers for others with terminal illnesses. "No one deserves to suffer like this." Her words repeated in my mind, urging me forward.

Stress was partially responsible for people falling ill, that was obvious, but it was not the whole story. In my research, I have found that wild animals were in constant stress of being eaten by other animals, and they were healthy. It had to have more to do with what was going *into* the body than with how the environment was affecting us.

My decision to listen to nature and follow her undeniable rules of creation was my first real step in my search for health. I became my own guinea pig, ready to do experiments on myself and become part of the natural plan of Creation. I was committed, and I started making plans.

Cleaning Out

I became interested in pH testing. I learned that one of the most basic barometers in the body, pH levels, reflect the acid/alkaline balance. Starting from a baseline figure that represents a good balance (it varies a bit from person to person), a test strip dipped in specific bodily fluids will reveal imbalances.

Without changing my diet at all, I recorded my numbers each day, discovering right from the start that I was dangerously acidic—the acids in my body were off the charts according to my test parameters. Testing for sugar and salt levels, I found them to be seriously imbalanced as well. I allowed myself to be honest, which was a little shocking, since I'd spent so much time denying my feelings. Now, although I continued playing the hard contact sports I'd always loved, I realized that no matter how well I looked on the outside, I was always suffering on the inside.

My ability to ignore my pain had gotten me through my mother's death, but it was no good to me now. I finally had to admit to my headaches; the pain in my feet, joints, and lower back; and devastating fatigue. On top of that, I had bad digestion, bloating, and severe consti-pation. My parents may have taught me to ignore physical pain, but I wanted the pain gone, and I was the only one who could make it happen.

I took some synthetic supplements at first, suggested by the people who turned me on to the pH testing. They thought I could restore the balance this way, but when I saw few changes and got nauseated to boot, I got tired of taking pills. I decided to attack my diet at the core and change what I was putting into my body daily. I had high hopes as I stopped consuming the enormous amounts of white sugar to which I was accustomed, but I had no idea how hard it would be.

I threw away the boxed cereals that were loaded with refined sugar, and I began to eat natural cereals made from wheat and other grains. They contained pasteurized honey, fructose, and other sweeteners, and I was still loading on extra honey and milk. My new breakfast was a far sight better than what I'd eaten in the past and I felt better at first—until the cravings began.

I compensated for these cravings by drinking large amounts of bottled fruit juices. They were not freshly squeezed, but they said "all natural" on the bottles, and I got them at a health food store. What was wrong with pasteurized fruit juices? I also drank 100 percent concen-trated juice in the mornings, since the advertising and the health books told me that it was perfectly fine.

As I dug into extra helpings of dried fruits, date sugar, bananas, and raisins to further satisfy my sugar cravings, I thought I was Nature Boy. Little did I know I was still consuming enough sugar, although in a different form, to aggravate my symptoms. But I was making other changes in the meantime, such as switching from white bread to whole wheat, from regular pasta to wheat and spinach pasta, and from potato chips and corn chips to whole-grain crackers and rice cakes.

I tried eating more dates—the health books said they were good— but they gave me tons of gas. I would walk around with a bloated stomach and terrible indigestion, feeling like I was pregnant, falsely secure that since I was no longer eating white, processed sugars, I was getting cleaned out. The trouble was that the supposedly healthy "all natural" bottled fruit juices that were supposed to calm my sugar cravings were part of the problem.

When I decided to eliminate "bad" food from my diet, I became aware of how much of my daily intake came from fast-food joints. It seemed logical as a college student to grab a quick burger or a taco from the nearest stand, since none of us had time to cook. But as I talked with my fellow students, I discovered that they were eating fast food from morning to night. Fries and onion rings, grilled cheese and burgers, sugary sodas and milk shakes were the fare of nearly every student with whom I spoke.

We had become a culture of fast and easy, with no regard for healthy. Since the early fifties, when the fast-food industry really took off, its advertising and marketing geniuses had turned around our culture, making this jaded way of eating seem normal. The conditioning was so effective that anyone who deviated was labeled a radical health nut. But the more people called me names and ridiculed me for bucking the system, the more determined I became. My health was deteriorating rapidly, my symptoms were getting worse, and I chose being ridiculed over ending up like my mother in the end.

For a long time, I focused on opening my bowels, since constipation was making me miserable. Hardened formations inside my intestines refused to loosen, and caused painful gripping attacks that doubled me over. I tried commercial laxatives several times, but they never worked well for me in the recommended dosages. Because I was such a severe case, I upped the dosages and suffered the gripping cramps that resulted. Even the instructions on the packages warned consumers against bad side effects from high doses of the medicine, but that was the only way it worked for me. After a great deal of pain and disappointment, once again I decided to abandon synthetics and go the natural route.

My first experience with natural herbal laxatives did not work that well, but at least I was saving my body from side effects caused by the toxins. On my own, I manipulated the dosages and hoped for results, while I continued to take the natural herbs that I believed would eventually clean out my body.

Carlos's Story

I had liked boxing ever since I was a kid, and although I was skinny, I was strong as hell and I kicked ass. While in college, I got back into boxing and kick boxing. I sometimes went to visit various gyms around town, to watch the guys spar.

One day I spotted a big Cuban guy named Carlos, who was standing next to the ring. He was about five-seven, with short, curly, jet black hair, but overweight, at about two hundred pounds, with a protruding gut that hung in folds over his trousers. His face was covered in acne so severe that his curly beard whiskers looked like they were trying to penetrate huge boils on his face. He had quite a mouth, and he cracked everybody up as he commented on the sparring, often with four-letter words.

I looked at nineteen-year-old Carlos holding a Coca-Cola in one hand and a couple of candy bars in the other. He popped some prescription meds for his ulcers and chased them down with a swig of Coke. The guy was a walking train wreck, but there was something under there that I liked.

"Maybe if you stopped drinking that crap and tried water instead," I blurted out, "you'd feel a hell of a lot better."

Carlos looked at me with interest as I continued. "In fact," I said, "if you detoxified and let all those demons fly out of your ass [he had no idea I was speaking from direct experience], your language might even improve."

He laughed and so did I. It was the beginning of an unusual relationship, and we liked each other from the start. I had no illusions about this crazy Cuban. From his rapid-fire expletives, I knew he was no saint, and from the looks of his huge, protruding belly and his exploding acne, I could see that he had health problems. I knew he was wild and unpredictable, but I could tell immediately that he had a heart of gold.

When we went out for a bite together, I found out how desperate he was and how much pain he was in. He was fascinated with my search for health, and while most people considered it radical and ridiculous, Carlos was entranced. He had been in pain for a long time, and he had never found a doctor who could help him. As we continued to talk, I found out that as bad as my foot condition, headaches, and digestion were, they were nothing compared to what Carlos had endured for so many years of his life.

When I heard he was scheduled for stomach surgery, I was not surprised. From what he told me, he had pain every time he ate, he'd been on over-the-counter antacids for a long time, and he'd landed in the emergency room for his ulcer pain more times than he could count. His severe stomach bloating was exacerbated by his obesity, and he had constipation, fatigue, headaches, and the worst acne I'd ever seen. He told me that not only did it go from his hairline to his neck, it also covered his chest and back, and he was too embarrassed to take off his shirt in public. The topical acne creams the doctors had prescribed did nothing. Neither did the prescription meds that he was swallowing constantly. In essence, the white coats had turned him into a walking drugstore at nineteen years old.

When Carlos asked me what I thought he should do, I asked him to tell me in detail everything he ate and drank from the moment he woke up to when he went to bed. I was thrilled to have a healing partner, someone who was willing to join me in my quest for health. I dubbed him Guinea Pig #2, and we were off and running.

I listened with horror as he described his diet. When Carlos woke in the morning, he would drink milk or Hawaiian Punch. Then he would eat Pop-Tarts, a Danish pastry, or jelly doughnuts. He always had candy bars in his pockets and there was always an open bag of Cheez Doodles, potato chips, or Frito-Lays in his car. I'd never seen him with anything but a soda in one hand and chips and candy bars in the other. Because he was overweight, he said, he tried to drink some diet sodas every day but he didn't like the taste, enlightening me about the large number of multicolored artificial drinks he would guzzle between the sodas. He was always dying of thirst. When I asked him how much water he drank, he laughed. "I don't need to drink water," he said, "'cause there's water in the Coke. Read the label."

Carlos told me that in high school, he would occasionally bring his own food to school or go to the 7-Eleven for a wrapped white bread submarine sandwich, a candy bar, and a Slurpee. This was a change from his usual can of soda. On other days, Carlos would run over to Burger King for a Whopper with extra cheese, or to McDonald's for a Big Mac, large fries, hot apple pie, and either a shake or a soda. When I asked Carlos why he didn't eat the lunches at school, he said they were boring and too healthy.

The typical school lunch was a riddle to us all. We never could figure out what we were eating because it was processed and covered with gravy. We called the main protein mystery meat, and the only way we actually knew what we were eating was by reading the menu on the cafeteria chalkboard or hearing it announced over the loudspeaker at school. Next to the mystery meat was a wad of mushy canned vegetables with no taste swimming in margarine. Next to that was a slice of cake covered with icing, or neon-colored Jell-O with canned fruit inside. And you had your choice of either a big piece of white bread or a roll and butter—or, should I say, margarine.

We often tried to stuff half of this disgusting, inedible food in a carton of milk. Even back then, our instincts told us that the mushy dead food on our plates was bad for us. I wondered who had set up our great food pyramid, which obviously was failing. No wonder the health of our country was so screwed up if this is what they considered a healthy and balanced diet.

My parents only gave Doug and me enough money to pay for lunch at school, prohibiting us from wasting their hard-earned money on fast-food joints and junk food. Why should we spend money if there was a reasonably balanced school lunch?

Carlos said he ate pretty much the same junk food for dinner that he ate for lunch, unless his mom got home in time from work to cook a huge Cuban family meal. Carlos and I ate basically the same foods at breakfast and lunch, and although my family cooked southern-style, the dinners at both our households were loaded with tons of grease, flour, rice or potatoes with gravy, all kinds of sugars, and lots and lots of bread. Dinner was followed with caffeine and desserts.

Carlos and I, both athletic by nature, began to compete with each other to regain our health, as we faced an uphill battle with very little support from the outside.

"It's not going to be easy," I warned him. I already knew that no one had a bag of tricks for us and that we needed to be patient, since natural food and remedies worked in their own slow but safe fashion. "We'll be working with Mother Nature on her terms, not ours," I explained. "We need to trust the process. I'm finding that out the hard way."

I wanted Carlos to understand what I had trouble accepting myself: there would be no instant gratification or quick fixes. That mentality, the quick-fix, instant-gratification syndrome, had to go out the window—we had to give up any thoughts of rapid changes.

Even as I explained how long it had taken me to get this far and how minuscule the shifts were at first, Carlos was impatient. "I don't have much time," he told me. Then he burst into a smile. "Maybe we could add some Cuban coffee to our diet, just to speed things along." I asked him to describe his physical problems in detail.

"Hope you have all day," he warned me as he began his list. "I'm a fat pig, I have excruciating headaches, my stomach burns like it's ready to fall out. I have bloating, I fart like a dog, I have a stuffy nose all the time, I have joint and back pain, I feel tired and wired, and I can't sleep. I'm anxious, I have either constipation or diarrhea. Shall I go on?"

I decided to start by pulling him off everything that had sugar in it, just as I had done with myself. He got excited and said, "Which things?"

When I started naming the foods and drinks that contained sugar, he nearly had a heart attack, since I had named almost his entire diet. "What?" he yelled. "You have to be kidding. There's nothing left for me to eat or drink!"

It was so much worse with Carlos than I ever expected. When I told him to drink at least four to six glasses of water a day instead of the bottled juices, he looked at me like I was from another planet. "Do I have to give up sodas?" he asked reluctantly.

"Absolutely," I answered. "They're loaded with sugar."

Panic spread across his face. "So what can I drink?" he asked.

When I considered all the sodas Carlos had consumed in his lifetime, I was reminded of the corrosion on the terminals of my car battery. The stuff had been so hard and thick, like a rock or a boulder, you couldn't knock or chip it off with a hammer and a screwdriver. My dad and a neighbor who worked on cars told me to pour a can of Coca-Cola on the corrosion and let it fizz. Then they suggested I use a toothbrush and scrub gently, and the corrosive rocks on the terminal would start to break apart.

I couldn't believe my eyes. As I poured on more Coke and just kept brushing, the rocks broke apart and fell off until soon it all was eaten away by the Coca-Cola, which literally burned and melted away the corrosion. After that day, I never drank another can of Coke again. Can you imagine what it does to a person's teeth? No wonder Carlos's stomach was burning and he had an ulcer at nineteen! If Coke can burn a hole through corrosion, what does it do to the delicate, soft tissue in our stomachs?

If Carlos conservatively drank 5 sodas a day, that added up to 1,825 cans of soda in one year. And it took one can of Coke to clean years of corrosion off my battery. It's easy to replace the terminals of your battery, but it's not so easy to replace your stomach.

When I further suggested that Carlos drink lemon and water when he got up each morning to clean out his liver and balance his pH, you'd think I'd read him a death sentence. When I was researching alternative cancer therapies for my mother, I'd learned that lemon and water made a powerful liver cleanser, while it also helped balance a person's pH.

Carlos asked if he could drink lemonade instead, to which I answered, "No."

When I saw him begin to panic, I made him a deal. "A half hour after the warm water and lemon," I bargained with him, "you can have orange juice from concentrate or natural juice from a health food store."

This calmed him down a little, until he asked me what I thought he should eat. When I described the foods I was eating—fresh vegetables, fresh fruits, and lean proteins—he freaked out, but he followed my advice.

His new breakfast consisted of eggs and a piece of whole wheat toast. At that point in time, I believed that was a healthy breakfast. I said he could have fruit instead of eggs if he so desired, and he looked at me like I was out of my mind.

For lunch, Carlos began eating chicken, fish, or meat. At nineteen, I didn't know all that much about good oils, but I did know enough to stay away from foods fried in batter. "Batter makes you fatter," I told Carlos. I recalled visiting my distant relatives in Georgia, where most of them were as fat as the pigs they raised. A great-uncle had patted his potbelly after a hearty dinner of fried chicken and mashed potatoes and said, "Don't worry, boy. When you're thirty or forty, you won't be able to see your toes, neither."

They laughed all the while they shoved white mountain cake, ice cream, and pecan pie into their ever-so-lovely, swollen cheeks.

I was on a steep learning curve as I continued to hit the books, study, and work the experiments on myself and Guinea Pig #2.

I told Carlos, "I need you to start eating fresh vegetables." I needed to eat more of them, too, as I showed him how to steam vegetables in water, not cook them in oil, as our parents did. Of course, Carlos hated eating steamed vegetables; they tasted bland to him, and he said he'd rather die than eat his veggies that way, even with the herbs I suggested.

He committed for a month and I felt that we were making headway, but his challenges were daunting as he began to withdraw from sugar.

I felt for him, I knew sugar cravings firsthand, but I also knew what would happen if he stopped the process.

For the first few days, Carlos had unbearable headaches as he fell asleep at night and then awakened to run to the bathroom to eliminate. He said he wanted to attack me physically every day. His agitation from sugar withdrawal was so extreme, he was exploding in fury. At noon on day three, he called me up, screaming like a madman.

"What's the emergency?" I wanted to know.

"I thought I was imagining it, but it's happened with every single meal and I'm freaking out. My stomach is *not* burning when I eat or after I eat. What's going on? I haven't felt like this since I was a kid. *¡Oiya!* This is un . . . be . . . *lee* . . . vable. Wow!"

He was blown away and so was I. We both realized we were on to something big. We were really excited.

By day five, Carlos wanted to stop taking his antacid and ulcer medications because he was no longer in dire pain. I didn't know what to advise him, since there was still so much I didn't know. By that time, the words with which I had been indoctrinated, "Consult with your doctor," would not come out of my mouth. I felt like I was sitting in the midst of a vast ocean with no land in sight, no compass, no radio, and a Popsicle stick for a paddle.

In two weeks' time, Carlos stopped his meds all by himself—something I do not necessarily recommend. The burning in his stomach never came back, and the tight knot that was gripping his stomach had loosened. It was time to introduce some herbal laxatives to his regime.

Carlos grinned when I suggested it. "Good," he said. "There's nothing like taking a good dump!"

I started him more gradually than I had done with myself, hoping to save him from the pain that years of constipation could cause. The truth was that he was happy throughout the process, calling me when he eliminated and describing shapes, colors, and smells—a lot more information than I needed to know. Ultimately, just those kinds of details have proved crucial to my research over the years.

At about this time, Carlos and I started noticing changes in his skin. The huge boil-type welts on his body and his face had stopped pushing out and were no longer forming big red pimples and whiteheads. His skin was starting to calm down a bit, and he was freaking out.

I told him to stop using the skin medication because I thought it was blocking his healing and actually pushing the poisons back into his skin. He agreed. "I stopped the ulcer meds and look what happened," he said. "My stomach started healing."

"You stopped the ulcer meds?" I said, growing alarmed. "Cold turkey? What are you . . . nuts?"

"Yeah. I stopped that medication. There was no way I was going back and start taking all that crap again. Those stupid doctors kept me on a load of crap and it never helped. My mom spent all that money and I just drank some stupid water, I gave up the sodas and sugar, and I'm getting better," said Carlos.

Creation made water, and man made Coca-Cola. Water is good for cleansing your body, and Coke is good for cleaning your car battery. Carlos canceled the stomach ulcer operation, outraging his doctors and frightening his mother, but he was feeling better every day. Why mess with success?

I began to log Carlos's changes so I could determine the eating patterns by which he and I had been victimized, only beginning to discover how simple it really was:

Water stopped his stomach form burning, so you could drink water. You could drink water even if the stomach was burning.

As the sodas left his body, Carlos loved drinking water, which cleansed many of his organs.

As the sugar began to leave Carlos's system, his energy stopped yo-yoing, and he gained a powerful sense of well-being.

As he stopped eating junk food and sugars, his acne boils began to disappear.

I was thrilled for him, but I also have to admit that as I observed the dramatic changes in my friend, I was frustrated that I was changing less rapidly. Only years later, I discovered that the sugar in the natural dates and figs I was consuming in large quantities was affecting my horrible foot condition. I had mistakenly replaced my addiction to processed sugar with an addiction to a more natural form of sugar, but it was still too much for my body to handle. Carlos, never a fan of dried fruits, had better results eating oranges and apples.

I was healing, too, although my changes were more subtle. I had more energy during the day, I didn't feel like sleeping after lunch, and my headaches were diminishing. The severe morning stiffness and knee inflammation were lightening up, and I could move from a sitting position to standing with much less pain. The constipation, however, had not improved all that much, and my feet were still flaking.

I continued the research, trying to figure out what was wrong, when many of Carlos's friends began calling me for advice. They were seeing his changes, they were amazed, and they wanted to talk with me, too. I decided to start working with other people to gain more knowledge of how they responded to this natural, simple system of eating and cleansing. I hoped to help them and I also hoped, through working with them, that I would get some answers for myself.

CHAPTER THREE

Indecent Exposure

My Uncle Bob called me one day to report that ongoing research was now revealing that pesticides like those we had used, such as Dursban, malathion, and chlordane, had severely damaging effects in the long run. DDT, another chemical we used, had been found to poison large animals in the food chain. It was so toxic, they were considering banning it, which they eventually did.

"Just imagine what it did to us," said Uncle Bob. "You, Cecil, Doug, and I have to be pretty poisoned by now."

Of course I agreed. Then he told me that Dr. Winston Jebson was coming to his home. Many years earlier, while working for NASA on the Apollo space program, Dr. Jebson had helped to develop a specialized camera with a highly sensitive lens that could read the most precise and subtle planetary color changes in subdivided areas of a photograph. Now he was utilizing the same technology to read disease histories in the irises of people's eyes.

When Dr. Jebson arrived at Uncle Bob's house, my brother, Doug, and I greeted him. "This camera," he said, "can give an in-depth tissue analysis and it can move past the iris to photograph the optic nerve." In

33

this way, he told us, he was able to detect weaknesses and profound body dysfunctions.

Only a few minutes after he looked into my eyes through his lens, he reported a dangerously high toxicity level throughout my body. "What have you been exposed to, Timothy?" he asked, with a troubled look on his face.

I darted a quick look at my uncle, who swore he'd told Dr. Jebson nothing about me or my history with pesticides. I told the doctor about the exterminating business.

Dr. Jebson nodded his head. "That explains it. I've never seen so much toxicity in a young man your age," he told me candidly. "You're so poisoned from heavy metals, it's a miracle you're still alive."

I remembered when all the kids on the block would run after the pesticide truck that was killing the mosquitoes, getting soaked in the toxic fog streaming off the back of the truck. I explained to the doctor how my brother and I had climbed under houses and sprayed chemicals for such a long time, we were covered in poisons by the time we got back out. I told him that I'd started helping my dad at age six, that huge barrels of toxic chemicals always sat in our garage in open vats, and that Doug and I had played around them.

Dr. Jebson began to rattle off my symptoms, which were frighteningly precise. "Not only are your liver and vital organs compromised," he said, "the heavy metal content in those pesticides could be trapped in your tissues and your large intestine is involved. Having any trouble with constipation?" He gave me chills, he was reading me so accurately.

Then he told me about a kind of testing called hair analysis to confirm the toxins locked in my body. I decided to send my hair sample to the lab, and I got back my results in the mail. Pages and pages of findings reported that my heavy metals, as well as my brother Doug's, were off the charts. I was initially alarmed and asked Uncle Bob if the lab could have sent us the wrong results. He wasn't sure, so I sent another hair clipping for a second analysis. In two weeks, however, I got identical results that reported dangerously high levels of arsenic, mercury, lead, cadmium, aluminum, and other heavy metals.

It was undeniable: I was severely poisoned. But now that I had the information, what could I do about it?

I showed my alarming test results to my hippie friend who worked at the local health food store. I respected his knowledge concerning health and nutrition, and he was his own best example, since he always looked so vibrant, a condition he attributed to eating mostly raw, live foods. He showed me one of his books called *Become Younger*, originally written circa 1920 by Dr. Norman Walker, the originator of the raw-foods movement. I bought the book and began introducing more live foods into my diet.

When I showed the guy from the health food store the numbers on my hair analysis tests, he said, "Wow! These are intense. You're having a couple of bowel movements a day, right?"

I was embarrassed to admit that I was lucky to have a bowel movement every second or third day. I thought back to when I was searching for alternative cancer therapies for my mom. Someone had recommended "colon therapy," more popularly known as "colonics." I decided to try it, and I managed to locate a colon therapist in Miami. Aware of how impacted my colon was, I was not looking forward to the procedure, since my large intestine was always jammed with rocklike feces. As the colon therapist slowly released water into my large intestine, trying to remove what was locked in there, despite my high pain tolerance from pushing myself as an athlete, it felt like he was stabbing me in the gut with a butcher knife. Unfortunately, the water didn't make it through the blockages, and I suffered extraordinary pain, but I came back for a second session.

When the same thing occurred, I decided I needed to find a way to get my bowels moving *before* I returned for a third session. I tried drinking small cans of prune juice—to no avail, since the fruit sugars wiped me out and put me to sleep. I went to the health food store to pick up a herbal laxative, but there were very few choices. I chose the strongest one I could find and decided that if the suggested laxative dosage was one tablet, I would take three. I was so plugged up, why not go for it?

I expected "things" would open up in an hour or so, but nothing happened. I decided to take three more. Maybe I hadn't taken enough. Or maybe the herbs were weak compared to drugs. If you know anything about herbal laxatives, I was taking straight senna leaf, which can be harsh if you take it improperly.

I was enjoying a gorgeous hot Miami day, standing at the park's entrance right beside my house when my intestine gripped so hard, I doubled over and fell to my knees. I couldn't stand, I could barely breathe, and I lay there, shaking and sweating, wondering if I was having an appendicitis attack. I was all alone, and when I looked over at my house, my front door seemed a million miles away. It was like being in a horror movie. I was unable to imagine how I would ever get to the house, while my sphincter let me know in no uncertain terms that getting to the bathroom was critical. My colon was boss, in charge of my every thought and movement.

I began to crawl slowly along the burning hot pavement, one hand on my gyrating guts as I made my way to my front door. I stopped every few feet as another wave of intestinal cramping doubled me over and I tried to catch my breath. Finally, when I had a minor release of cramps, after I said a big prayer, I tightened my sphincter and bolted for the bathroom door as all hell broke loose.

I sat on the toilet for hours while what felt like boulders and water streamed out of my bowels. It went on like that for the rest of the weekend as I drank water between mad dashes to the toilet. I was pleading with my colon to be my friend, while it was letting me know that my abuse had gone too far and our relationship was about to change.

By Sunday, two days in, I looked outside and noticed that everything seemed more vibrant and greener than before. I was exhausted, but at that moment I felt better than I could remember feeling in years. I felt like I had released at least fifteen years of toxins from my bowels. I decided to take a modified amount of laxative before my next colonic to make my life a little easier. The colonics were still massively painful, but at least the toxic material was finally starting to move out of me. My colon and I agreed that we would build a new mutual relationship built on respect from then on.

After two powerfully intense series of six colonics each, I needed to figure out how to bring out the more deep-seated toxins. I turned to something natural: psyllium husks. They didn't work at first, since I had no idea I was supposed to drink tons of water with them, and I got even more constipated, but I kept at it. For a while, I was so bloated I felt like a beached whale walking around, but when I modified the amount and started to flush it with water, things began changing in subtle ways.

Realizations were coming to me constantly. The more aggressively I worked to remove toxins, the worse my symptoms raged, from headaches to cold sweats to joint pain to fevers. When I look back, I wonder how I got away without killing myself in the process. I attribute it to using natural formulas, because if I'd taken the equivalent amount of drugs, I probably wouldn't be here to tell my story. It was trial and error, and I broke all the rules before I found out what they were.

The fact that I always felt better after the detoxes kept me going. I had to keep reminding myself that nature worked in its own time, not mine, which wreaked havoc with my tree-cutting business. I'd be on a high branch, a rope wrapped around my waist as I worked the chain saw, when suddenly I got a bowel attack. I looked down with envy at my two employees on the ground while my large intestine revved up.

During this trying, painful time, I thought back to how every doctor I'd ever seen had assured me that my flaking feet, excruciating headaches, and constipation had nothing to do with what I was eating. They were wrong, dead wrong, and only when the pain eased could I appreciate how toxic my body had become and how necessary this painful cleansing process really was. I would see it through, no matter how bad it got, but I prayed for healing every day as I struggled to change my lifetime of habits that had landed me in such an unhealthy state.

One day, I got a phone call from my dad, who was in a small hospital in Georgia, complaining of severe abdominal pain and about to undergo surgery. I begged him to wait until I got there, and I boarded the first possible plane. The trouble was that he feared he had appendicitis. The doctors did nothing to quell his fears and by the time my plane landed, my dad was already in the operating room.

After the surgery, I watched him lying unconscious as I sat there in disbelief, praying. It looked like my hero was dying, and I could do nothing to help him. I couldn't even get information on the surgery they'd just performed.

The next afternoon, his doctor walked in while I was there, and I was all over him. "What did you do to him and why?" I wanted to know. "Did he have appendicitis?"

"No, he didn't," the doctor said.

"Why did you operate, then?" I asked. "What did he have?"

"Well," the doctor stalled for time, "we aren't really sure, but we suspected cancer so we removed a third of his colon."

When I asked to see the tissue biopsies to confirm cancer, the doctor ignored me and walked out of the room.

My father languished in serious condition for days on end, a huge, gaping scar across his abdomen. I later learned that he had nearly died during surgery because the doctors had not drained his bowels properly before the operation, as they were supposed to do. As a result, peritonitis and toxic shock nearly killed him. Now that I had seen the results of my own poisoning, his had to be the same or worse. Two weeks later, my dad was released from the hospital. His health was permanently compromised, but at least he was alive.

My dad was back home, and it was about six months after my buddy Carlos had changed his diet. The changes he had continued to undergo were phenomenal, as his stomach had healed to the extent that he had no more burning, his headaches were gone, and his previous inability to concentrate was a thing of the past. Most profound was the healing of his skin. The boils had not only stopped multiplying, the existing ones had dried and disappeared. We thought that he would have to live with large pockmarks on his face—that could not be avoided—but when the quality of his skin started to change and many of his pockmarks started to recede, we were blown away.

Needless to say, Carlos was ecstatic. His weight loss (forty pounds in five months) stunned his friends, and so did his posture, as he had begun carrying himself as if he liked who he was. I had to keep reminding him that his miraculous healing had happened because of his commitment to himself and to the process. It took that degree of determination to get the kind of results he was enjoying.

When I considered the big picture, I came up with a car analogy. Why were our cars giving us great mileage and a good ride while our bodies were losing steam and breaking down? The answer was that we maintained our cars according to the way the manufacturers had designed them. We brought them in for checkups, we changed the oil, and we fed the car the fuel it was meant to burn. When it came to our bodies, though, we did *not* maintain them according to how our Creator had designed them. We didn't slow down when we felt tired, we lost sleep that was crucial for regeneration, and we did not feed ourselves foods that our Creator had designed for us.

The upshot was that we took better care of our cars than we did ourselves. Had our fast-paced "quick fix" lifestyle gotten us into irreversible trouble? Human beings were supposed to be the most evolved species on earth, with the highest intelligence. If that was true, why were most wild animals, plants, and insects healthy and thriving while we were not? What had happened to our instincts and common sense? If caring for our bodies was meant to be simple, the secret to good health had to be good maintenance and following correct lifestyle patterns. In other words, it was simple but not easy.

When I started to review what had worked so well for Carlos, it was now obvious that he had been severely dehydrated for years. Carlos's stomach burning and his ulcers were instantly corrected with water. What a simple solution! I pored through anatomy and physiology books to learn that our blood plasma is primarily made up of simple water. As a matter of fact, three quarters of the body is made up of water, and every single day of our lives, our bodies require a particular amount of water to function—to live.

The more water that Carlos and I drank, the better we felt. We realized that water was instrumental in washing toxins away. It also made sense that if dehydration caused toxins to become superconcentrated, then our bowels, liver, and digestive organs needed water to flush themselves out. As Carlos and I drank fresh water and ate pure food, we were eliminating not only the toxins, we were also eliminating the causes of our illnesses—the object of my search ever since I first decided to change my diet and my life.

I fantasized our medical doctors looking toward causes instead of dulling symptoms with quick fixes, charging an arm and a leg for drugs, and moving on to the next patient. Imagine what would happen if they stopped prescribing Band-Aid–like medicines such as aspirin for headaches? What if instead of prescribing drugs that kept the toxins locked inside our bodies, they told us to "drink lots of water and call me in the morning"? That kind of commonsense thinking could actually ruin their business. No wonder they were so dedicated to keeping things the way they were.

With Carlos's healing and my own following close behind, I was determined to continue down the road I was on to see where it led. I was still somewhat constipated even after a dozen colonics. I had some more cleansing to do. As Carlos's friends started approaching me for advice, I had my guinea pigs all in a row. Unbeknownst to me, this was the beginning of my private practice. With each person who came to tell me his or her story, I was building a growing, thriving, ever-changing practice that was more like a think tank, since I wanted the client as involved in the healing process as I was. I'd always been interested in instincts and common sense, I was open to everyone's ideas and participation, and that attitude has continued to this day.

The Miracle of Enzymes

I had reached a point in my research where I determined that disease could not exist or survive in a truly healthy body. My mother's body had not been healthy, because she had eaten so poorly throughout her life. Neither was my father's body, as a result of exposing himself to processed and refined foods, smoke from fires, alcohol, and pesticides. Now look what was happening to him. The question was, what caused the body to become unbalanced and therefore unhealthy? Alternately, what created a healthy, balanced body?

I turned back to Dr. Norman Walker's books about eating raw, as I added more raw foods to my daily intake and more information to my insatiable brain. Dr. Walker stressed how essential it was to chew food well. If we chewed until it turned into a liquid form before swallowing, he said, we could break the digestive enzymes out of the cell walls and properly digest our food. Fascinated by the miracle of enzymes, a totally new concept to me, I found extensive research on the topic compiled by the scientist and researcher Dr. Edward Howell. I loved studying his comprehensive information on enzyme production and metabolism.

Contrary to the more current popular theories, Dr. Howell's theory, "the adaptive secretion of enzymes," was based on simple scientific data. He explained that the body has a finite number of *metabolic enzymes*. These enzymes are key to our health and life force, as they help produce the energy needed for our bodies to function properly. Dr. Howell contended that each bodily function, from eating to sleeping, from walking to reading a book, was made possible through access to the metabolic enzyme bank that literally "ran" the body. He believed that if we used up our enzyme stores, just like closing out a bank account by removing the money, we would die.

Dr. Howell named three specific types of enzymes: metabolic, digestive, and food enzymes. Again, as with opening different bank accounts for saving or checking as needed, we have access to different enzymes that are produced as we need them. For instance, digestive enzymes are produced when we need to digest. At the same time, sensors in our mouths signal the body to create food enzymes we might be missing when we eat cooked food in which the enzymes in those foods have died.

I considered the enzymes inherent in every plant or animal food. According to what I now understood, our foods were bestowed with a specific amount of enzymes needed for proper digestion. If you cooked food up to temperatures between approximately 106 and more than 119 degrees Fahrenheit for more than a few minutes, the inherent enzymes died. Then we had to mobilize and steal enzymes from our own body's metabolic reserve to produce enzymes that were destroyed in the cooking process so we could digest. The more we stole, however, the more we wiped out our reserves.

Dr. Howell wrote that grains, seeds, and nuts contain enzyme inhibitors. It was only when water hit the grain, seed, or nut that it would activate. Then we could digest them properly. He talked about the value of sprouting grains and seeds in water before eating them, warning that if we didn't, the enzyme inhibitors would require our bodies to produce a huge amount of enzymes to break down that nut, seed, or grain.

Dr. Howell contended that enzymes were temperature-sensitive and pH-specific, as each enzyme became active only in its designated pH range. If we killed the enzymes by cooking the vegetables, grains, seeds, nuts, and meats, we were relying on our own precious enzymes. If our systems were not in that particular balanced pH range in which enzymes became active, they wouldn't work properly.

In fact, every enzyme is pH-specific and will work only if the pH is within normal range. The ramifications were staggering when I considered that many of my clients ate almost exclusively cooked foods with dead enzymes, relying on their own body's enzymes. It was no surprise they were bloated and tired and had indigestion as they devoured refined sugars, breads, pasteurized dairy products, candy, and sodas as well as highly cooked meats and fats. According to daily pH tests, these foods were turning their bodies acidic and creating imbalances. Many of the enzymes needed to digest these foods could not be activated. In other words, our miserable eating habits had completely screwed up our pH ranges—when all we ever had to do was follow Mother Nature to keep our ranges in balance.

Digestion begins the minute you put the food in your mouth. The salivary glands in your mouth start secreting enzymes while you chew, and if you don't chew until the food is liquid, it won't break down enough for the next phase of digestion. Imagine your body trying to accept chunks of undigested foods. They could either pass out of the body in small, undigested pieces, or those pieces could stay inside your intestinal tract or your blood, putrefying and causing toxicity along with a host of other problems.

I was horrified when I watched people chew their food only a few times before swallowing. How did we expect to get the nutrients into our cells, organs, and tissues if we didn't chew properly? I recall Carlos taking a humongous bite of a burger and sipping his Coke before he finished chewing—once or twice.

When he changed his diet, disciplining himself to chew properly was a real challenge. I discovered that it took thirty to sixty chews to turn a food to liquid. I liked calling the teeth "the pearly gates to heaven," because they unlocked the nourishment to feed our heavenly and divine bodies within. Once the food passes the pearly gates, you could create either heaven or hell inside yourself—and most people were a living hell inside.

People's eating habits were, more often than not, breaking the laws of creation by eating cooked foods and processed food with no enzymes, not bothering to chew, and drinking freezing cold and hot drinks with meals, thereby diluting the food enzymes as well as deactivating them. Imbalances in our pH caused our digestive enzymes not to work properly. Many times it takes more energy to break the food down than we get from the food. This is why we stay tired. We have a real energy loss.

The situation is this: We cannot digest sugar and carbohydrates in the absence of the enzymes called *amylase* and *pitilyn*. For fats, we need *lipase*; for proteins, *protease*. If we constantly oversecrete those enzymes by eating foods such as sugar, bread, and cooked and processed foods in which the enzymes have been destroyed by the cooking process, we must secrete a compensatory amount of enzymes to digest that level of food. We then deplete our enzyme bank, which is why you can't eat the same foods at forty that you could at eighteen.

Where would I find other pieces of the puzzle?

Pasteurization and Homogenization

One day I found some information by Dr. Paul Auster, an expert on pasteurization and homogenization. He explained that the high temperatures required for pasteurizing dairy products not only killed enzymes, they also created a poisonous chemical called xanthine oxidase (the XO factor), which went directly into the arterial system and formed plaque. Alarms went off in my head. Heart disease caused by hardened plaque in the arteries had risen dramatically across the country over the past hundred years. So had our intake of pasteurized dairy products.

Dr. Auster went on to say that milk pasteurization killed a vital dairy enzyme called lactase. We were not able to produce it ourselves, and without it, it was impossible to break down the lactose. I cut out all dairy, even though it was a mainstay of my diet, and after only a few days, I awoke one morning with no congestion. I could breathe through my nose for the first time in years. The fissures on my feet started to diminish ever so slightly as well. Nothing had ever affected them positively before, and I was also thrilled to discover that my bowel activity was taking a positive turn.

It seemed like the circulation in my arms and legs was improving, as they stopped falling asleep so much. All this from eliminating cheese and milk? All I could think about was that advertisement slogan, *Milk does a body good!* Maybe raw milk or breast milk does, but pasteurized dairy doesn't. I wondered how many serious health problems Louis Pasteur was responsible for. After all, the marketing of pasteurized milk was another commercialized indoctrination by an industry that created health problems for our nation.

My challenge was to convince my clients to give up pasteurized cheese and milk—and therefore pizza—because raw dairy was illegal to obtain. No one wanted to give up these things, except clients with the most debilitating allergies who were willing to try anything for their constant congestion, sneezing, and profuse postnasal drip. When they cut dairy out of their diets, most of their symptoms cleared up and their problems disappeared.

Some of my clients had spent thousands of dollars taking allergy shots for years, completely overlooking the simplest solution. Cut out the pasteurized dairy and you can breathe again. Here was yet another lesson from God: *Eat it the way I created it!*

. . .

I had just graduated from the University of Miami when I decided to move to Southern California, where the health movement was thriving. I arrived in Hollywood with an army bag and four hundred dollars in my pocket, and I hooked up with my old grade school buddy, Roy Sekoff, who already had moved to West Los Angeles. We became roommates, I pounded the pavement for work, and in two days I landed a waiter's job at Bono's Restaurant.

I was so broke back then, I often worked double shifts while I continued to detoxify my system in every way I could find. I fasted and I got something called a "colema board," a personal colonic system that enabled me to do something like a colonic on myself, in the privacy of my own home.

I cleansed aggressively and continued working double shifts while the pesticides literally flew out of my body. As I cleaned out my intestines, a horrible, smelly, rubberlike substance poured out of me, and I felt more and more vulnerable. One day I had a powerful impulse to call my father to tell him how much I loved him. I did not understand the urgency of the feeling as I dialed his number in Miami.

"Hi, son," he said, as a lifetime of bottled-up emotions came rushing into my throat.

I finally managed to say, "Dad . . . I just wanted to tell you how much you've taught me. And I wanted to thank you for everything you've done for me, for my whole life." After what felt like an eternity, I got out the words I'd always wanted to say. "I love you so much, Dad."

My dad composed himself and said, "I love you, too, son."

Two weeks later, my dad had a heart attack and died. His life was cut short because his body had broken down prematurely, something that could have been avoided with knowledge and practical application. I was stunned, and my world crashed.

On the day of the funeral, I learned a great deal about my father as I spoke to people who had known and loved him. His life had been all about helping others, and despite a brutal childhood, he had positively touched hundreds if not thousands of people's lives.

Following the ceremony, two of my dad's friends called him the sweetest and most ethical person they had ever met. I thanked God for allowing me to follow in my father's footsteps by helping people, one person at a time. It was easy to get discouraged with a medical system that would not let real healers heal. It seemed that threats to big business were considered a crime. But I knew in my heart that great health was the birthright of every human being, and I refused to sit back and watch greedy industries take that right away from us.

I remembered a conversation with my dad before my mother died. "Son, you have so much passion and fire," he'd said, "but you don't understand how corrupt the system is. Nothing we do will make a difference a hundred years from now—no matter how hard you try to change it."

I refused to accept that, and as I looked around the room at all the people whose lives my father had changed for the better, I realized that he hadn't accepted it either. Each kind act he did added to his legacy of service. A hero to many, my father would be my role model now, as I worked to continue his legacy. I felt it was the least I could do, as I gathered the courage and conviction to stand up tall in the name of my father and unconditionally support the things in which I believed. I was ready to return to Los Angeles, and with my dad inspiring my path from his well-earned seat in heaven, I would bring to light the truth about God's creative healing force.

CHAPTER 4

Curing the Incurables

When I returned from Miami to Los Angeles, I felt like someone had stolen a piece of my heart. I was restless and deeply unresolved, filled with regret that I had not made it back to Miami for my dad's last Christmas. I realized that both of my parents had died prematurely because of their toxic lifestyles, and I didn't want to repeat their patterns. I stepped up my detoxifying process. Although they had done their best, my parents had next to no nutritional information, and with each bite of food, they had slowly and silently been killing themselves.

Refusing to go the same deadly route, fasting was the next logical step for me. I continued using my colema board as well. During that time, while I was fasting and doing colonics, Roy would walk into the apartment we shared and hold his nose. He was appalled by the stench of pesticides, so much so that he thought an exterminator had come by to spray when he was out. I had only to inhale the atmosphere to know that the terrible poisons were finally leaving my body. The doctors had been wrong again. It had taken this long and this much cleansing to get to the pesticides, and now the stench filled the apartment. For days on end, we had to keep all the windows open to air it out.

As I continued, the deep fissures in my feet finally started to heal. In three to six months after I began fasting, my feet looked completely different, and I remembered the doctors' declarations that I would never heal, that I would have to live with these problems for the rest of my life. They also had said that the pesticides and my diet had nothing to do with my condition, but they were wrong again. There was a simple solution, I had found it, and I was ecstatic when I saw the changes, although they left me with more questions.

I was bewildered that when I fasted, the skin on my hands and feet was moist and soft, a far cry from the fissures, flaking, and intense dryness. But when I started eating again, the soft, moist skin would dry up. What in the world was making this happen?

I was sharing a pound of dates with Roy one afternoon, each of us farting our butts off as we sat on different sides of the couch, when the lightbulb turned on. I stared at the deep bowl filled with pits on the coffee table and I had one of those Aha! moments. The dates, figs, and raisins I was devouring daily had to be the causes of my present imbalance. No matter that they were organic, natural, or anything else. The water content had been eliminated in the drying, which concentrated the sugar content. Although I'd given up sugar in its refined form, I was still consuming more fruit sugar than my body could metabolize.

Since the sugar was feeding the fungus in my body that had taken over my feet, it made sense that when I stopped eating it, the fungus starved and my feet healed. When I started eating sugar again, the dryness returned because the fungus was being fed again. The answer was right under my nose, or more accurately, it was in my mouth as I was removing the cause.

Incidentally, when Roy saw what I was doing, although he had never cleansed or fasted before, he jumped on the bandwagon. Along with eating raw food like I was doing, he began taking intestinal cleansers five times a day. In a short time I was amazed to see his lifetime allergies and his stomach problems disappearing.

Nine months after I'd moved in with Roy, I found my own place nearby, on Gateway Boulevard in West Los Angeles. There I built my own personal health laboratory. I felt as if my father were urging me forward as I got everything I needed in the area of bodily biochemistry testing equipment, as well as germinating jars, for sprouting, juicers, raw fruits, vegetables of all sorts, and jar upon jar of herbal formula experiments. I had turned into a mad scientist, I loved every second of it, and my friends were fascinated as they started calling me the sproutologist, the rawologist, the juiceologist. Their favorite name for me, though, was the professor of everything.

I was still numb from my father's passing when my car was rear-ended by a drunken man who was driving more than sixty miles per hour on a city street. Suffering a severe back injury, I was bedridden for months, during which time I read everything about nutrition I could get my hands on.

Tired of lying flat on my back and not agreeing that I needed surgery, I found Franco Columbo, a chiropractor and bodybuilder with a different approach. While others advised me to do no physical activity whatsoever, Franco believed that the inactivity had only prolonged and worsened my back injury. An outside-the-box thinker, he suggested ways to rebuild my atrophied muscles, in combination with taking my herbal formulas. In a short time, my back injuries began to heal, and I felt well enough to restart my nutritional practice. With a great deal more research under my belt, I was eager to see the clients I'd missed so much during my months of inactivity.

My practice was growing fast, and my office was filled with medical rejects—the hardest cases, the "incurables." Working with people in so much pain forced me to dig deep into their roots to discover the causes of their imbalances. I always began by taking extensive background information, including as much information as possible about what they ate and drank from the time they were born.

Patterns emerged almost immediately, and I was soon able to tell people what was wrong with them just by analyzing their diets. I usually knew which enzymes they had overexcreted and the imbalances that resulted. From studying iridology, sclerology (reading the eyes), dermatoglyphics, and their symptoms such as bodily signals and weaknesses, these patterns led me to an understanding of their underlying imbalances. I also relied on my own intuitive analysis based on repeated family patterns, lifestyle, and diet. People thought I was psychic, but I was simply using common sense, a good commodity in the healing world.

Todd's Story

As I took on the cases that the doctors had rejected, I met Todd Bryant, his condition a medical mystery that had earned him a place in the ranks of the incurables, a term in which I did not believe. A good friend of mine who knew Todd took me to see him, and we all sat on the lawn outside his house to talk.

Todd was a strapping guy, about six-two and 175 pounds. He was young, blond, handsome, and rugged, with a powerfully ripped body that made other guys jealous. I liked the guy right away. He appeared to be a disciplined, professional athlete, but I noticed that his breathing was labored. When he took one of his inhalers out of his pocket and sprayed it into his mouth, I was taken aback, not by what he was doing but by the fear in his eyes. I encouraged him to tell me his story.

Todd had been gasping for air since he was young. All he'd wanted was to play with his friends, but he spent so much time doubled over, desperate for oxygen, that his parents took him to a doctor. The pediatrician gave him an asthma diagnosis and prescribed Marix, an anti-wheezing medication that helped the constant wheezing somewhat. But he was still being rushed to the emergency room with major asthma attacks. The hospital would inject him with Adrenalin and shove an oxygen mask over his nose and mouth. It took every bit of strength he possessed to squeeze the tiniest bit of oxygen into his lungs. After what seemed like an eternity to him, Todd's bronchial tubes started to open and he could breathe normally again. These frightening incidents scared the living daylights out of him; and why not? He couldn't breathe, and he was traumatized, always dreading the next episode. That was the fear I had seen in his eyes.

During his teenage years, his condition worsened, which prompted his doctors to prescribe more drugs. He started using steroid inhalers that opened his bronchial tubes immediately but left him with severe headaches and heart palpitations. The palpitations often got so bad that he had to bend forward and wait for his dizziness to pass. He abhorred the side effects from the steroids, but he needed to use them or he would die—or so he had been told. As a result, he had two inhalers with him at all times and several more in his car and at home. When he told me he'd been forced to find a place to live near a hospital so he could get to the emergency room when he had attacks, I wondered how he could live such a nightmarish existence.

When he graduated from high school, Todd was fed up with never being able to exercise. He wanted to be active and strong like everybody else, and he joined a gym, only to discover that any kind of cardio exercise initiated a series of asthma attacks, sending him straight back to the emergency room. I asked him if he had ever tried to get rid of his inhaler.

"Yes," he said. "I tried for a while but it really didn't work." It seemed that for no apparent reason (not apparent to him, anyway), he was suddenly back in the emergency room with the worst attack ever. It took so long for his lungs to open and for him to breathe that he almost died. Once he got back home, he'd been frightened sufficiently to stop his own experimenting, and he started back on the drugs consistently. Todd became visibly excited when I told him about my own health problems and how I had turned things around.

"All my life," he said, "I've been praying for some real help with my 'incurable' asthma. Will you work with me?"

I saw the frustration and exasperation in his eyes. I was hooked, and I agreed to work with him.

I'm sure it's no surprise to you that I explored Todd's diet first. As with almost everyone, he would have to change it completely, but he was willing to suffer the changes for a modicum of relief. I immediately took him off all cheese, milk, and other dairy products that were mucus-forming. He went on fresh juices, he agreed to do cleanses, and the first fast was really hard on him.

He told me how tough it was to drink juices and water all day, then sit down in front of the TV at night to relax and be tortured by junk food commercials. Literally swallowed up by advertising, he craved a Big Mac, a sloppy cheeseburger from Burger King, and most of all, pizza. Todd missed pizza more than anything, but he felt so much cleaner and could breathe so much better without it, he stuck with the process.

I was happy he was staying strictly on the diet, but there was a great deal more work to be done. I read a book by Robert O. Becker, M.D., and Gary Selden, *The Body Electric*, and I gained an understanding of body electricity. I also found another book, by Dr. C. Samuel West, *The Gold Seven Plus One*, in which I learned that we need to keep the electrical current alive at all times, communicating between cells. When the electricity gets interrupted, cells start to die rapidly. To maintain that electrical relationship, cells must be tightly touching each other so the current can jump back and forth, a situation called negative subatmospheric pressure or the dry state. If too much fluid escapes the cell and surrounds it, the cells separate and electrical communication stops. The subsequent loss of electricity at the cellular level ultimately leads to cell death.

I sought out this highly informed man at a health convention I attended, where he was promoting his book. Without going into the detailed science behind his discoveries, he was able to speak to the layperson. "The simple act of jumping up and down on a minitrampoline and breathing deeply," he told me, "can radically change the electrical relationship between cells."

Dr. West said that when a person jumped into the air and reached the highest point, during the split second when he began to come back down, gravity was reversed. At that point the trapped fluid surrounding and between the cells got washed away. The cells could then come back together naturally and resume their normal electrical conductivity.

He went on to describe specific factors that helped keep the polarity of the cells in a balanced state, such as raw foods, live juices, acupuncture, and herbs. Conversely, sugar could interrupt the electrical cellular polarity. It became clear that a large part of Todd's problem was a serious fluid buildup in his lungs and bronchial tissues. My idea was to keep the electrical current in a balanced state while he removed the fluid from around his cells, along with all the trapped poisons and toxins.

Todd bought a minitrampoline, and while he began jumping his way back to health, I devised herbal formulas to support his particular imbalances and specific body weaknesses. I knew it was vital that Todd become "remineralized," especially during this intense detoxification process. I advised him to juice celery and dark leafy green vegetables, and thanks to his dedication and compliance, he was starting to see results.

It was gratifying to watch Todd's excitement when after only two weeks into his new regime, he noticed slight improvements in his breathing. A short time later, unbeknownst to me, he took a radical plunge and went off his inhalers, cold turkey. I've never suggested that a client do anything cold turkey, and I would have advised him against it, which may have been the reason he didn't tell me. When I found out, I was worried about him, but I secretly believed that deep healing would never occur as long as he kept pumping his body full of steroids, the so-called medicine in the inhalers. Common sense was leading both Todd and me as he made his individual decisions and I stood behind him.

After the fact, he described to me his trepidation when he first tossed his inhalers into the trash can. After all, he was as indoctrinated as the next guy when it came to drugs, and he still went to doctors for antibiotics to heal infections from time to time. But the more he stayed on his new path and embraced my philosophies, the more he learned to trust his body as his best healer. He came to his own conclusion that drugs didn't heal anything, that all they did was suppress the problems more deeply. I finally understood that drugs not only suppressed the real problem but also set the stage for greater imbalances, problems, and possible diseases.

Within six months of being off his medications and staying faithful to my protocols, Todd was making huge progress. These days, when he had trouble breathing, he reached for a glass of fresh celery juice instead of an inhaler. The results were not as immediate as with an inhaler, but he was slowly learning that if he drank the fresh green juice and relaxed, his lungs would open up and he could breathe comfortably. He'd stopped having asthma attacks when an interesting thing began to happen. Each morning when he woke up, he coughed up huge clumps of hard, smelly, yellow mucus, some of it black inside and hard as rocks.

"What do you think is going on?" he asked me.

I thought a moment and then answered, "I think these clumps of mucus have been in your lungs for years." It was logical that the hardened stuff had been caused by the mucus-forming foods he'd eaten and all the drugs he'd consumed his whole life. His body had been producing the mucus for years, so where could it go? "Your body couldn't get rid of it fast enough," I said, "and your lungs became a repository for it, just like the pesticides stayed in my body. But you're expelling it now, bro."

"Is it okay?" he asked, concerned that maybe he was going too far.

"It's very okay," I said. "You just let it come up. Your body knows exactly what it needs to do."

Todd continued to cough up hard yellow clumps, and each day he felt better. He stopped wheezing, he became virtually asthma-free, and he was beginning to take deep breaths as he continued to expel mucus over the next seven years. His heart palpitations subsided, and he was able to run four miles with no breathing problems. His dream had come true. Todd's "incurable" asthma was gone, never to return, and he left the ranks of the "incurables." After dedicating himself to healing his body with the help of Mother Nature, he became an athlete after all, working as a professional stuntman for movies and television. I couldn't help but marvel at the human body's ability to slowly heal and reorganize itself, given the opportunity. Todd cured Todd.

That was all Todd did (it was all I did, too), and our bodies began to steadily find balance, the natural state to which we all would like to return. Once again, I had seen that nature was the only real healing key, whatever the problem. Today Todd Bryant, athlete and stuntman, is living, breathing proof of that.

A Macrostudy

Guided by simplicity and common sense, I was slowly unraveling the mystery of optimum health. With each new piece to the puzzle, I realized we'd been *conditioned* to believe that health was a mystery. It wasn't, and I became inspired, applying my research theories about water, sugar, live food, enzymes, and pH balance.

The looming question was this:

What was key here—what we were doing wrong or what we were not doing right that created our problems? I hung out in my ever-expanding health laboratory, with experiments being conducted in every corner of the apartment. You could barely take a step without falling over herbal formulas, germinating sprouts, whirling juicers, and colema boards.

During the time my mother was dying, I'd read about the eating system called macrobiotics and the insightful Japanese man named Michio Kushi who had introduced this Eastern concept to the West. Still, I had some reservations, since Michio Kushi's opinion on "raw vs. cooked" differed from my own. He believed that sick people could not digest raw foods. I disagreed, aware that if someone chewed food to its liquid state, the enzymes would be released and would make the food easily digestible. And yet I was impressed with how macrobiotics positively affected a person's pH balance.

The more I read, the clearer it became that the macrobiotic principles were aimed at one thing: *creating balance in the body*. It was about eating foods that came directly from the earth. Here we go again, I thought with a smile. Back to nature. All the reputable health pioneers, no matter their particular systems, were talking about the earth's wholeness and the avoidance of processed and altered foods and drugs.

The macrobiotic diet emphasized eating grains only in their whole form, and was extremely supportive of eating cooked brown rice. White rice, pastas, cereals, and breads were prohibited, considered to be denatured and destroyed, along with all other grains that had been polished, bleached, or starched. The proponents of macrobiotics agreed with me that there were next to no original nutrients left in the "white stuff," since the refining process altered, damaged, or killed what goodness had initially existed in the grain.

What about whole grain bread? I wondered. Was that okay?

I was still eating grains because they claimed to be "whole." But they weren't really, were they? In fact, by the time the original whole grain had been processed into bread, it wasn't a grain anymore. I thought about the refined flour products I'd been consuming all my life—the bread, pasta, tortilla chips, and hamburger buns. Even after I'd changed my diet, I still ate whole wheat pasta, whole grain breads, rolls, and organic tortilla chips made with nonhydrogenated oils. And I thought I knew my stuff! Well, I may have been doing a lot better than some of the other people I knew, but I was missing the boat, big-time. I was still constipated a lot of the time, and so were many of the people I knew. I had only to turn on the television to see that the number-one over-the-counter medication in this country was laxatives. The bottom line was that no one could easily defecate in America, one of the most healthful, enjoyable, affordable forms of entertainment!

With a commitment to try macrobiotics, I cut out all my beloved whole grain breads and pastas and began to eat sprouted cooked brown rice, even though everything else I ate was raw. I eliminated without the help of herbal laxatives, uncommon for me at that time, and I rarely if ever felt my energy drop quickly after a meal that contained brown rice.

Now I understood that with the whole grain breads and pasta I had eaten previously, the sugars had released into my system too quickly because the fiber was no longer in its original form and because the rest of the whole grain was then ground down into flour. I also found that if grains were not sprouted, we would have an adverse reaction because the phytase in the grain was not releasing the phytic acid. Our body then recognized the incorrect form of this food as a foreign invader.

I started thinking about the popular viewpoint that buzzed around the nutrition world, calling these whole grain bread products "complex carbohydrates." There were whole books written on this subject that reported carbohydrates to be a necessary part of our diet. That was true. But after these grains were turned into flour, they weren't even close to their original complex form. They released more like a simple sugar, which was way too fast for our bodies to metabolize and burn. The fiber in these bread products was now broken down compared to what was originally in that whole grain to begin with.

I realized it was just a stripped-down, pale copy of what it had originally been. With refined grains of any kind—white, whole wheat, oat, spelt, millet, quinoa, rice, corn—if they were altered in any way and turned into flour, they became detrimental to our bodies. I decided to use sprouted brown rice as a transitional food for sick clients who were heavily addicted to flour products.

Furthermore, I was learning that refined grains were a huge factor in the deterioration of our bodies at the cellular level, especially when we ate them consistently. They couldn't be metabolized fast enough, and when not used up, they fermented inside the cell, creating acidity that forced the oxygen out of the cell. This was true whether a person ate white or whole wheat bread, spelt, or organic corn tortillas.

Here's how I broke it down:

- Incomplete metabolism of sugar created fermentation.
- Fermentation forced oxygen out of the cell, causing cellular asphyxiation.
- Cellular asphyxiation led to havoc and death at the cellular level.
- Oxygen starvation at the cellular level created a fertile ground for cancer to grow!

I realized that we, ourselves, were predominantly responsible for creating oxygen starvation at the cellular level because of our incorrect eating and drinking choices.

What a simple answer! If I was discovering this on my own, where was the medical community? They were supposedly looking for a cure for cancer. I did not find out until some years later that in 1931, a man named Otto Warburg won a Nobel Prize for discovering that cancer could not live in a highly oxygenated body. Wouldn't you think that this might be a path to follow if you were *really* looking for a cancer cure? Otto Warburg had discovered that cancer would grow in an anaerobic, or low-oxygen environment. But as I worked with all my sick clients, I realized I was discovering the actual incorrect eating patterns that had created the conditions for a low-oxygen environment to exist. In other words, in my opinion I was learning how to remove the *cause* of cancer. If the medical and pharmaceutical industries claimed to be looking for a cancer cure, why weren't they looking for the factors that were creating the cause?

My clients and I began to eat cabbage, cruciferous vegetables of all shapes and sizes, daikon radishes, and an array of seaweeds such as kombu and hijiki, crucial parts of the macrobiotic diet. The sea vegetables in the diet contained a uniquely broad spectrum of nutrients that were many times greater than those of land vegetables. We followed many macrobiotic-suggested menus, and I even gave the nod to a certain amount of sprouted cooked brown rice, a food that seemed to round out the entire program. Yes, we were all eating a little sprouted brown rice at first, a complex carbohydrate in which the whole grain prevented the sugars from being released too fast, thereby avoiding an oversecretion of insulin. I mostly stayed off it, though, since I felt best eating only raw foods.

There was just so much to learn! I decided that whatever was good and would benefit my clients I would use, and whatever did not work well, I would discard.

From reading other great works, and from working with my clients, I had some idea about how important it was to keep the fluids of the body in balance. But how did one really achieve this? I remembered that the body was made up of about 70 percent fluids and that our bodies were created similarly to the earth. About three quarters of the earth is covered with water, and a great majority is covered with seawater. Of the elements contained in our bodily fluids, I wondered how closely proportionate those elements were to those of seawater. I knew that our bodily fluids needed to stay in a specific proportion of macro- and microminerals and other elementals to maintain balance. From all I had seen so far, it seemed that the macrobiotic diet was helping to do just that.

I thought back to what I had learned from Dr. West about the importance of the lymphatic system. I remembered his brilliant teaching about blood proteins and fluid escaping from inside the cells. When these fluids escaped, it would cause excess fluid and sodium to become trapped around the cells. This could cause an imbalance between the potassium and sodium inside the cell. As Dr. West stated, "Anything that will upset the sodium-potassium balance can damage or kill the cell."

This was crucial because it was the sodium/potassium pump and the rotation of sodium and potassium in and out of the cell that generated an electrical field. We know that every cell is an electrical generator, so the energy produced by the cell must be the key to the life process. When the cells lost fluid, they lost electrical communication, they lost their own electricity, and they died. I couldn't forget that we lived in an electrical body, one of the critical factors that determined life or death at the cellular level. Dr. West had discovered a certain formula for life and a formula for death at the cellular level, theories he presented to Professor Arthur Guyton, who wrote *The Textbook of Medical Physiology*. After a bout with polio, Guyton became chairman of the department of Physiology and Biophysics at Oxford University. In his famous textbook, written in 1947, he stated how important it is to have our bodily fluids in balance.

The recurring theme of balance was always in play. I recalled a multitude of doctors who clung tightly to their beliefs that even with a critically ill patient like my mother or my father, their diet had nothing to do with their debilitated condition. Had they ever thought about the balance of nature? Did they even read their own textbooks? They obviously were making up science as they went along, but where did they expect the nutrients to come from—pizza, soda, and their prescription pads? There had to be a way to renourish and rebuild our body fluids daily.

As I used Dr. West's great information in my work, and as my clients were recovering faster, I became hungry for more knowledge. I needed to make sure my clients were eating a diet rich in nutrients, but how did I know which elements were present in their bodily fluids and how much they used up each day? Were they getting enough nutrients from their daily intake of food? If not, what would happen to their bodies? How could they possibly be getting enough nutrients if the soil was poisoned and not rotated, which killed the microorganisms that delivered the nutrients to the plants? We were now eating pathetic plant life. It was obvious that we were not getting what we needed. What was a body to do?

Man-Made vs. Nature-Made

I read about a brilliant researcher named Alexis Carrell, who kept a chicken heart alive in a petri dish for twenty-five years. His experiment started on January 17, 1912. Apparently simply by changing the fluids every day and keeping them fresh and balanced, the little chicken heart did not age and remained in perfect condition. It died only when Mr. Carroll went away and his assistant forgot to change the fluids one day.

If only we could change our own bodily fluids and feed ourselves the right nutrients and minerals. Instead, we do the opposite as we spend years out of balance until all our bodies can do is struggle to stay alive. In the end we lose the battle, and that is when our degeneration becomes obvious. My mantras, day and night, were two questions:

How do we maintain the balance of our bodily fluids? How do we replenish them constantly?

I considered what I thought the correct balance should be, and what proportions needed to be maintained. I discovered immediately that the range of needed elements was vast, and they needed to be replaced continually as we used them. There was no way we were getting what we needed in our diets, and as always, Mother Nature had to be the answer. But how could I find replacements for the bodily fluids that had not been manipulated and depleted by man?

I turned to Guinea Pig #1, myself, for research experiments, since I was still suffering the effects of my early pesticide exposure. I was getting a new piece to the puzzle now, with my study of macro- and microminerals, as well as electrolytes and elementals, both known and unknown. Dr. Walker had stressed that drinking live juices was one way we could get some of the missing minerals and other nutrients we needed.

I started juicing like crazy, making sure to dilute the fresh juices with water to lower the sugar concentration, which was too high. The juices gave me an immediate sense of well-being and vibrancy as I fed my body a quicker and more broad-based range of electrolytes that helped my electrical body. The more I drank, the better I felt, and so did my clients as the daily hum of juicers in their homes announced they were juicing their way back to health. Unfortunately, though, as helpful as this was, my clients were still not getting a broad enough mineral range. I had more work to do.

In my clinical practice, I returned to the very important topic of pH ranges and how they were affected by the lack of elementals in the system. If a client did not replace the used elements constantly, his or her pH would fall dangerously out of balance and the client would get sicker and sicker. The pH needed to remain constant, staying within a tight margin and always needing to remain in a homeostatic balance. It didn't matter what their symptoms were. I noticed that if I continued to feed their bodies all the needed elements, they would eventually come back into the correct range and start to get well.

I was feeling a big difference in my own health, but a person can only drink so much juice! There had to be another way to replace those missing elements. My clients and I tried the mineral combos they sold in bottles at the health food store, but they tasted metallic and did not feel right in our bodies. It was all about man-made vs. nature-made. Whenever I took something man-made, it tasted metallic and I felt bad. In contrast, when I took herbal formulas or natural foods, they tasted great and I felt alive. I surmised that real food sources automatically contained the macro- and micronutrients in proper balance along with the cofactors on which minerals depended. In the same way, real food sources also contained the proper amount of water and enzymes that delivered minerals to the tissues. Man-made minerals could not compete with this kind of synergy.

My clients and I were off and running as I took them off all breads and flour products, allowing them only sprouted grains. We all consumed a great deal of raw, living foods, which were so easy to digest, we rarely felt tired. We juiced ourselves, did massive detoxes, and got healthier by the day. I stepped up making my herbal formulas for congested and deficient organs, fully aware that we needed to be renourished all the time. I devised my formulas individually for each person, according to his or her body weaknesses.

I continued my seven-to-twenty-one-day fasts and cleanses every seven weeks. I pushed myself hard and I was racked with intense pain as my body threw out years of heavy metals and other toxins. I recall lying in a warm bathtub in absolute agony one evening, praying to God to either take me right then and there or get me past this bump in the road immediately. I got through it and now I see that as much as I suffered, those radical cleanses saved my life.

Now that I was living alone, my apartment exploded with herbal experiments. I dived in with both feet, gathering together every bottle, jar, and health contraption I could find. I was getting the most difficult cases, and it was stressful, as I was running by the seat of my pants. I had my books for research and my test results and those of my clients to educate me and help build my theories, but nothing could have prepared me for what was coming my way.

CHAPTER 5

Kathy's Story

I had met a couple named Lenny and Nancy some time back, and Lenny had experienced a major healing breakthrough. It was customary for a satisfied client to spread the word about me, but when Lenny told me someone named Kathy would be calling, I had no clue what I was getting into.

When Kathy's kids were very small, her husband was killed in an automobile accident. Since then she had been a single mother, supporting her three children all by herself, struggling to keep her head above water. Recently, when she was wondering how she could keep it up, her worst nightmare happened. She was diagnosed with breast and colon cancer, and given a death sentence by her attending doctor. In fact, he told her, her cancer was spreading so quickly he didn't know what they could do.

Kathy was grief-stricken. What about her children? What would become of them when she died? As it was, she could barely put food on her table, and she had no support system—no family and no backup. During her first visit to my apartment, she sobbed and moaned over and over, "What am I going to do? What am I going to do?"

She looked at me with such unbelievable anguish in her eyes, I panicked. She was looking to me for answers, for hope, for a solution to her misery. I felt like bolting straight out of there and out of Los Angeles altogether. I had never worked with anyone who had cancer. As she talked about her situation, visions of my mother surfaced, and I really had no desire to get involved with that kind of desperation. She continued to beg for my help, so I decided to listen to her story—the least I could do.

I watched Kathy carefully and listened well as we spent the next three and a half hours together. She was thick-bodied, with gray, pasty-looking skin. Her huge abdomen was abnormally distended, and she was in constant pain. Now, with a diagnosis of multiple cancers and only a few months to live, she had to keep working so her kids could eat. When she told me she had been severely constipated all her life, I nodded. But she was in worse shape than I had ever been. Over the years she had taken her problem to doctors who ran tests (something they were very good at) and told her she had nothing to worry about as they took her money and gave her prescriptions for laxative-type drugs that only made matters worse. Finally she got so discouraged, she stopped seeing doctors altogether.

When she found blood in her stools and a breast lump, however, she went back to the doctor because she knew she should. Accustomed to being the Rock of Gibraltar for her kids, she wasn't really worried—until her doctor told her she had terminal cancer. He might as well have shot a hole in her heart, she told me, because she was so surprised. She went home with a terrible secret, since she could not bring herself to tell her children that she didn't have long to live. And now here she was, sitting in my living room!

I had no idea what to do for Kathy. Where would I even begin? I was in my early twenties without information or experience in this sort of thing. I dreaded a future with more people like Kathy knocking at my door, and I went to bed that night praying to God that she would not call me in the morning. I had no way to handle her problems, and part of me wished she would somehow disappear. Instead, she called, I answered, she called and called and called, and we set out on a terrifying journey together.

I started by reviewing her history, which informed me that all her life, Kathy had been the Bread Queen. She had literally lived on bread products almost exclusively, eating muffins and pastries for breakfast, sandwiches for lunch, and pasta for dinner. True, it was quick, cheap, and easy, but it also was deadly. I figured if she wanted any chance at all, even to buy a little time, she would need to radically change her diet. I immediately took her off all flour products, the most difficult change she would have to make. I made sure to add sprouted brown rice to her diet, since I expected difficulty when she went off the flour products that had made up most of her diet for most of her life. Then I waited, hoping she would have at least enough time to figure out how to set up her children when she died.

Kathy continued to awaken each day panicked about her children and how to provide for them, wondering if they would end up homeless and then in an orphanage. I worked in the meantime to ease her intense cycles of pain as I tried to take pressure off her severely compromised system. I thought I knew where to begin, but I had to be extremely vigilant about keeping her changes slow and gentle. With so many toxins lodged in her colon and the rest of her system, if she dumped them too fast, I was risking sending her into toxic shock.

My task, once she agreed to change her diet, was to open up her bowels as quickly as possible. Judging from my own experience and that of many of my clients, I figured that some bowel cleansing would lessen Kathy's extreme fatigue. Also, I had her take a pH test. Her saliva and urine pH ranges were so off, Kathy was essentially a walking bag of acidity!

I used my knowledge and experience to make natural formulas for her that would lubricate and soften her bowels. She alternated the formulas every few hours, even though she went to work every day. I recalled the start of my own bowel cleansing, and I didn't envy Kathy one little bit. But the fact remained that her bowels simply had to open up, and finally, open they did!

As I had suspected, her first bowel movements were so hard, she was in agony. She increased the doses of my lubricating, softening formulas and changed her diet. Needless to say, she missed her Danish pastries in the mornings, eating a small helping of fruit instead, which took some getting used to. And she continued to take the formulas I concocted for her daily. I worked carefully to make sure she didn't get any debilitating intestinal griping, since she told me she had a history of spasms in her descending colon.

Her first morning at work with the formulas in her system was uneventful. In the afternoon, however, she called me, complaining of a fever and a headache. No matter how gently I had formulated her herbs, she was so filled with toxins, her fever was spiking. Even when it reached 104 within a few more hours, I did not panic. I knew in my gut that this had to happen, that her body was heating up to mobilize white blood cells to usher out the toxins. I recalled how it had felt when my own fever had spiked like that—the feeling that my head would surely explode at any moment as I lay in the bathtub, wishing for a quick death so the headache would disappear. I knew that detoxifying an extremely toxic system was not pretty but necessary, and I advised her to keep cold compresses on her head and continue taking the formulas, which, to my amazement, she did.

Every hour on the hour Kathy called me, checking to see if her terrible symptoms were normal. Once, she called her medical doctor, who had told her the headaches were signs of a massive infection and prescribed antibiotics. I knew he was trained to prescribe drugs, but I believed in the inherent wisdom of the body, that it had a reason to heat itself up to create the enzymes needed to go after the poisons and the rest of the invaders. I believed that introducing antibiotics to stop the process would be the worst solution of all. Thank God Kathy agreed with me, because as is always the case with my work, all final decisions I left up to her.

A day and a half had passed without a bowel movement for Kathy, but I knew something had to give if she could just hang in there. It was two full days later when her bowels opened, releasing a movement that was so hard and impacted it caused her excruciating pain. She went forward anyway, and I lent her a juicer and taught her children how to use it so she could have fresh juices around the clock. Kathy's bowel movements softened each day, and the more fecal matter she passed, the more her fever came down and her headaches lessened.

On day four, she called to tell me she had never eliminated like that and she was actually feeling a lot better. The pain that had plagued her body was diminishing. That sounded fine, but I was at a loss, challenged like never before. I had only been trying to give Kathy some pain relief and maybe buy her some extra time to find a home for her kids. Now that she was feeling somewhat better, I had no idea what to do next for her. I prayed for answers each night before I fell asleep, and Kathy continued to take my intestinal formulas and put in a full day's work.

I felt compelled to make fresh green juices every day because Kathy was so busy, there was no way she could spend her time juicing. I admired her courage, as she never missed a day of work or caring for her children while she just kept putting one foot in front of the other, downing her formulas, drinking her green powder drinks, and going to the bathroom—all day, every day.

After ten days of a diet change and constant ingestion of herbal formulas, Kathy's pH range had begun to register on the pH test strip. I was stunned that her biochemistry was shifting so fast, and I started her on a liver/gallbladder flush to clear the way for a huge colon cleanse I had in the works. The flush got excruciating, as she was awakened in the night with so much pain on her right side, she called to tell me about it. She got scared because she was nauseated and had vomited and she called a half hour later to report no change.

Then, twenty minutes later, when I picked up the receiver again, groggy and worried about her, she had good news. In fact, she sounded happy as she explained a pulsing in her liver that had caused her to run to the bathroom, where she had a large bowel movement. "When I looked in the toilet," she squealed with a little too much enthusiasm for that time of night, "I thought the Jolly Green Giant had dumped a huge bag of peas in there. There were so many," she effused, "I couldn't even see the water."

Gallstones were flushing out of her gallbladder, a process that continued for the next two hours. She kept me informed every twenty minutes or so, as I gave up trying to sleep and cheered her on. With each bowel movement, she felt better. I was not surprised when I asked if her doctor had ever mentioned gallstones, and she said no.

After the release of her gallstones, I suspected Kathy had kidney stones in there, too, so I formulated a bladder and kidney flush, which she also took with no complaints. Now I was making formulas for Kathy all day and night to soften her organs enough to dump the poisons she had been retaining. When the kidney flush also produced results, her pain was diminishing, and we both felt encouraged, although we were also both completely exhausted from lack of sleep.

Now it was time for her to start the seven-day cleanse that I hoped would make all the difference. She took the various formulas I created to begin a deep cleansing process of her colon. That included getting on the colema board twice a day, during which time she continued to call me in agonized pain, in the middle of the night. It started at about 2:30 A.M. almost like clockwork, with messages that went like this: "Ooh, Tim, call me right away. I am in so much pain . . . can you please call . . . ooh . . . please call!"

I died inside each time the phone rang, as my stress levels escalated like never before. True, it had been terrible being awakened by my mother's sobbing all night long. I'd hated it, but she was my mother. How on earth had I gotten myself in this situation with Kathy, someone I'd only just met? It was a crushing responsibility to be her only hope—her lifeline. I was too young for this, I thought. I needed support, too, and I wanted to run, but there was no one to call and nowhere to go. I started begging God for answers, turning my faith to the healing power of His Creation. Then I continued to put my theories to the test. Could a deathly sick system recover if the internal environment were nourished, cleansed, and rebalanced? I was about to find out, firsthand, what God's creations were really designed to do.

While Kathy dumped a huge amount of hideous-smelling material from her bowels, I made her a lymphatic formula and asked her to jump on a minitrampoline five times a day. I was opening all the detoxification pathways, and she was drinking a ton of water and eating 70 percent raw fruits and vegetables. She went off all meat, she occasionally ate some seared fish, and I made my first formula specifically designed to support the body in dealing with cancer.

Kathy continued to call me in the night even as things were improving. I was such a light sleeper and got so accustomed to her middle-of-the-night calls, my poor, ragged nervous system would wake me up before the phone rang. I was like a man with a new baby, and it went on for months, until one particular night. I awakened as usual a little before 2:30 A.M., but the phone never rang. I waited a few moments and fell back to sleep.

In the morning, I awakened thinking what a beautiful morning it was—until I realized that Kathy had not called that night. I jumped out of bed and starting pacing. *Oh, my God,* I thought, *she must have died. What am I going to do?*

I picked up the receiver and dialed her number with trembling fingers, dreading what I might find at the other end. My heart was racing when she calmly said, "Hello?"

"Kathy," I muttered, "is that really you?"

"Who else did you think it was?" she teased.

I dragged the phone all over the room, dancing and jumping up and down.

"Tim," she said, "you sound out of breath, like you just came back from a run."

All I could think to say was, "Kathy, you have no idea."

As one day rolled into the next, I noticed that the more Kathy cleaned out her colon, the more the cancerous lump at the top of her right breast became angry and irritated, pushing its way outward. One day it turned yellowish-purple and began to open up and ooze thick, bad-smelling pus.

The old-time herbalists' teachings, where I turned for answers, were confident about the healing power of herbs. My own experience had created the same confidence in me, and I racked my brain to come up with a poultice I could lay on Kathy's cancerous lump that would pull toxins out of her tumor. I began making powerful herbal poultices (you could smell them a mile away), and Kathy wore them for hours at a time. When we pulled them off, the smell of rotting, decayed tissue combined with the odor of green and yellow pus was overwhelming! And still, onward we trudged, as she was ingesting and wearing an enormous amount of herbal combos at one time. I admired her fierce determination, and I kept her on tons of formulas and intestinal cleansers for the next three months. Neither of us wanted her bowels to back up like that again, and frankly, she could not ever allow that to happen.

I was on a mission to oxygenate Kathy's blood, so I added an oxygenating herbal formula to her regime, putting it into a liquid form so she could assimilate it easily. This was when her biochemistry really started to shift. When her pH strips became greenish, I literally jumped for joy at this encouraging indication that her body fluids were becoming balanced.

Kathy started taking walks in the sunshine and visits to the ocean with her kids. She followed my advice to do deep breathing exercises to oxygenate her blood, and she was feeling happy and hopeful. A miracle was occurring as she felt the life streaming back into her previously destroyed body. She was alive, she was looking to the future, and it appeared that she was defying her death sentence. Only time would tell.

I reviewed Kathy's changes and her continued efforts. She was doing cleanses, eating 70 percent raw, juicing, taking green formulas and many others, using breast poultices, and jumping on the trampoline. She had given up all flour and sugar, along with processed foods as she ate directly from the earth, sitting at Mother Nature's dinner table. She was doing everything she could, but she still feared for her children.

"Tim," she asked me over and over, "do you think I'm going to die? Am I out of the woods yet?"

"I don't know" was all I could say, because I didn't know. I refused to give her false hope and I kept praying for her, since I saw that her life was truly in God's hands. But things were really looking up, as her bio-chemistry became more balanced, her headaches were gone, and her breast lump had stopped oozing, become much smaller, and was drying up and scabbing over. She also had dropped fifteen pounds (that was never her intention, but she was overweight), and her distended abdomen was flattening. Over the next months her lump would disappear completely and she would go from an original weight of 170 pounds down to a healthy 118 pounds. My hope was that if she followed the natural order of Creation's design for us, her body would fully embrace its potential to realign itself, and illness would be a thing of the past.

Back to the White Coats

When Kathy's friends Lenny and Nancy, the couple who had introduced us, saw her for the first time after several months, they were stunned at the radical change in her appearance and her spirit. They wanted to know if her cancer was gone, but since I had no facility to run tests or do biopsies, there was no way I could say for sure. I had every intention of helping her heal, but I was worried that she was too far gone. I simply wanted to allow her body to do what it wanted to do naturally, and in my humble opinion, it was doing a mighty fine job!

In six months, Kathy felt really good. She had never deviated from her healthy regime, and in nine months she felt fabulous. She believed that the death sentence the doctors had read her was slowly being shredded by her body's own healing abilities. It had been about thirteen months. Maybe it was time to go back to the white coats, have a biopsy and some other tests, and get some confirmation.

The office manager was so stunned when she looked at Kathy's face and body, her jaw dropped. She figured this patient had died a long time ago, since she had stopped coming to see the doctor. The doctor's face turned pale when she walked in, and he looked like he had just seen a ghost. Even though it was obvious that he was stunned, he never mentioned her glowing state of health or bothered to ask what she had been doing. He didn't even say he was glad to see her. He simply examined her breast and scheduled her for tests and a biopsy.

A few days later, when the results came in, she got a call from the office manager to come back in immediately. "Something went wrong with your tests because your cancer disappeared and that just can't be true. We have to retest you again."

Kathy was tested one more time, and her results came back the same. No cancer cells. When she called me, she was screaming with joy. "The cancer is gone!" she said. She also told me that the doctor had shown no emotion whatsoever until she tried to tell him about me, our work together, and all she had done to heal herself. Threatened and furious, he ridiculed her, telling her that herbs and cleanses could not cure cancer. She had shouted at him and stomped out of his office, but really, her unadulterated joy could not be thwarted. Her nearly dead body had healed itself and now she had proof. She marveled at the miracle of Creation, and she now felt solid, alive, and grateful, filled with a hard-earned determination to live the rest of her life in harmony with nature. I could not have received a better gift. (For natural cancer prevention and therapies, see the resources section at the back of this book.)

I said good-bye to Kathy a few months later, when she moved with her children to the mountains. Now that she had a new understanding of how to care for herself and her family, she wanted to be closer to nature, living a life as free from stress and illness as possible. I knew that as yet

I did not have a full understanding of the amazing healing that had occurred in Kathy. What I did know was that as each client brought me the next piece of puzzle, it was starting to form a clear picture and an obvious direction.

I certainly wasn't prepared for the next phone call I received, from an attorney asking me if I knew Kathy. The doctor's attorney proceeded to tell me that if I didn't watch myself, I would get thrown in jail for practicing medicine without a license. I asked this attorney what constituted "practicing medicine without a license." I assured him that I wasn't using any drugs, I wasn't diagnosing or making any claims. All I did was change her diet and make her some herbal formulas.

Then I asked, "Is her doctor having you call me because she got well? Do they want to know what I did, or do they just want to scare me?"

The attorney became agitated, continuing to threaten to have me thrown in jail. By now, though, I refused to be intimidated by his empty threats. I had done nothing illegal, and I would be willing to say that in any court of law. "All I know," I told him, "is that she got healthy. If that's a crime, then have me arrested."

The attorney went silent. His anger exploded as he threatened, "You better watch yourself," and then he hung up on me.

All I could do was smile inside and think that I must be doing something right.

CHAPTER 6

Creation, the Real Healer

When I looked back at my work with Kathy, I counted my blessings. God had allowed me a glimpse into the amazing power of healing as I encouraged her to live by eating only what nature provided. In the end, it was clear that Kathy had healed Kathy simply by living according to the rules and laws inherent in creation.

When I understood for sure that Kathy had cured Kathy, I knew that the human body had the power to heal almost any disease. I'd been given the opportunity to face cancer, the monster of a nightmare that had caused utter devastation in my house, my uncle's house, and those of so many others. I had to realize that along with everyone else, I'd been conditioned by the medical industry to live in fear of cancer, which they labeled a mystery about which very little could be done. The experts considered cancer practically a death sentence, and Kathy had been given little hope for survival by her M.D., who deemed her condition terminal.

Thankfully, we had other ideas. I was astounded and awed, and after dealing with Kathy, I was never again afraid to take on anyone's condition, no matter how bad their doctor said it was or what they named the disease. I continued to apply everything I'd learned with each new client about regaining and maintaining optimal health. It turned out that no matter what they named the disease, the disease could *not* live in a healthy body.

Why did the medical industry come up with names for the conditions or diseases they could not figure out how to solve? Couldn't the public see through it?

A patient would see a doctor with a specific ailment. If the doctor couldn't suppress it and remove it, he'd give it a name and make it sound scary. Then he'd advise the suffering person to shove the symptoms down with a drug, all the while speaking about the illness as if it were a mystery. "We're looking for a cure!" these doctors would assure their patients. But I had yet to see them cure or solve anything they'd named a disease. Of course they couldn't cure it or solve it, because they rarely if ever looked for the cause.

This appeared to be the medical/pharmaceutical way—the habits of a couple of very successful industries. As long as they could keep the problem a mystery, they could keep a hell of a business booming! Nature, however, had something different in mind, and that was where I put my faith when it came to real health.

So far, in every single person with whom I worked, I noticed a recurring theme—no man-made food or synthetically manufactured drug inventions could touch the powers of Creation in its ability to support the healing processes that could lead us back to health. Creation alone could provide the real building blocks for the human body—Creation had its own built-in construction crew who knew more about the body than anyone on the outside ever could.

I continued to observe that the more deeply and consistently my clients applied natural principles, the healthier they became and the better they felt as their symptoms would slowly disappear. And eventually the disease would disappear, too.

This was so fascinating to me, I began slowly to rethink and research the entire premise of disease as well as "germ" theory. Based on witnessing my clients' healing processes, and compared with how nature worked, the currently accepted disease and germ theories were highly suspect as to their validity. It was clear to me that the drug industry, the very people to whom we looked for validation of man's systems, had created the concepts of disease and germ theory in the first place. They'd made up their own rules for linear, compartmentalized science in the application of drugs. But how could we consider such systems valid when we were still suffering from so many health problems and diseases? It didn't make sense.

I observed that every known disease continued to escalate, even after widespread treatment with drugs. If you turned to creation for real answers and building materials for the human body to regain health, you faced a monopoly created by the medical and pharmaceutical industries to stop anything outside of their system. In Kathy's horrendous situation with her so-called disease that they named cancer, in the end, creation had cured its own creation.

In other words, *you are the cause and you are the cure.*

Genetic Nonsense

When I returned to the very beginning of my own health problems and those of my family, the pieces of the puzzle seemed to be taking form, giving me a picture of the real answers to some of our problems. I reviewed my earlier cases, linked patterns, and saw clearly how most of us had created our own patterns and problems from a lifestyle of unbalanced choices. Most of us had created our own unbalanced internal environment. But where did we learn it? The answer is a simple one: our parents. That explained why certain health patterns and diseases happened to run through the same family.

When the doctors can't figure out how to get us well with their drugs, they say, "It's genetics—it just runs in your family."

Dr. Weston Price was a dentist in the early 1900s who dedicated his life to studying traditional diets around the world. He found that the cultures that ate crude diets directly from the earth in their raw form (including animal protein) had better health. The more civilized the culture became in its eating habits, the higher the mortality rate, and the more the cranial structure deteriorated and narrowed. It was obvious that cultures that ate processed sugar were not adequately feeding their bodies, having to steal minerals from their own bone structure to survive. This, in turn, affected future generations.

Let me propose this. If it were genetics, why was it that when I took my patients off the junk they'd been stuffing down their faces for a lifetime, their so-called genetic illnesses disappeared? Once they changed their eating patterns and took my herbal formulas, they healed. If it were really genetics, then no matter what they did, they would not have been able to reverse their conditions. If you are born with Down syndrome, correct eating patterns can support but never eradicate the challenge. That, my friends, is genetics! But when your doctor calls the incorrect eating and lifestyle patterns that have been passed down through your family lineage genetics, they're leading you down what I call the road to genetic confusion. It was clear to me that most weaknesses that were passed down from generation to generation came from the family table, a clear departure from what we have been conditioned into believing.

You have a choice. You can continue to repeat the same incorrect eating and drinking patterns that your parents passed down to you, which created the problems in the first place. If you do this, you feed the predisposition for these weaknesses until eventually you will create the same problems. It is not the gene's fault. The gene didn't eat and drink the thing that created your problems.

The other choice is to stop the bad patterns that your parents passed down, and refuse to feed the problem. You can start eating and drinking correctly and rebuild the underlying weakness. Then the so-called family genetic health problems will miraculously disappear. Your new decisions and actions will break the genetic ignorance that has been running in your family for years. You are powerful!

It's as easy as that. You can change your course of history, and you will no longer have to fear the diseases that run in your family.

If we have genetic predispositions for certain body weaknesses, if we heal and regenerate our bodies, we make it better for the next generation. I discovered throughout my work that genetics were a minor component of poor health compared with what we were facing in lifestyle and eating patterns. It didn't matter whether you called it sickness, unhealthiness, disease, or anything else. It was all about eating and drinking the wrong things over an entire lifetime. When I linked the causes of my family's problems, I saw that inadvertently we had each created these problems for ourselves.

I decided to work backward with myself, taking an honest look at my symptoms, my organs, and the integrity of my tissues. What had been locked inside this body of mine? Why were all the members of my family so sick? What laid the groundwork for so many imbalances to occur in the Brantley clan? What was our eating and drinking lineage? My mother's mother was obese and had died of diabetes. Type 2 diabetes is no mystery when you consider the fact that my grandmother ate sugar and flour products. What a family tradition, I thought, but it was similar to almost everyone else's. No wonder we were all ailing and weakened. Our bodies never had a chance.

My grandmother ate large amounts of refined sugars and refined grain products, and her table was set with starchy foods and sugary beverages. She fed her children a diet of highly cooked oils, and she fried and overcooked the meat until it was browned and well done. What did this do to her body and to her family's bodies? This kind of diet, rich in refined sugars and refined grains, forced the pancreas to overwork, causing an oversecretion of insulin. Considering the fact that my grandmother ate that way, as did all of her children, their pancreases were constantly overworking to secrete insulin. I could almost see the smoke rising from this tired little gland in my mother and my father.

Imagine putting brand-new tires on your car and burning rubber at every block. Very soon your tires burn out, which was exactly what had happened to my grandma's pancreas, the reason she became diabetic. The overeating of sugar overworked and tired out her pancreas. The highly cooked oils and fats she consumed regularly acted like a sheet of plastic covering her cells. She had gotten so clogged, even if she *had* been creating enough insulin to balance her blood sugar, which she was not, the insulin would have a hard time entering the cells this way.

My mother had been taught by my grandmother to eat and drink a certain way. Because my mom had followed her mother's example since she was a child, she craved unhealthy food. She called it comfort food, which she, in turn, fed to her own family, thereby continuing the pattern of eating white sugar and flour products from sunrise to sunset. If it was good enough for her mother, it was good enough for her and her children. This is what I call passed-down patterns of ignorance.

I still recall nights when I would watch my mother lovingly make dinner for our family. There she stood at the kitchen counter, melted Crisco sputtering in the pan, white flour all over the counter, as she rolled chicken in batter before frying it a golden brown. While she cooked, she was in the habit of eating spoonful after spoonful of raw chocolate chip cookie dough from a huge bowl. Who didn't overeat back then? Even if she had decided to bake the chicken instead of frying it for a healthier meal, it was still cooked southern style, which meant it was steeped in Crisco or cooking oil laden with trans fats.

My family believed that if we ate margarine instead of butter, it was healthier. At least that was what the advertisements said, but little did we know that consuming margarine would set the stage for chronic health problems. Were we ever sold down the river by the food industry!

Each morning when Mom woke up, she downed a cup of coffee with tons of white sugar. Then she would stuff down a Danish pastry, maybe a Pop-Tart or two, a doughnut, and a bowl of cereal with extra sugar on top. While she fed us cereal and Pop-Tarts, she'd be shoving toast with margarine and jelly down her mouth until she finally sat down and said, "I'm not hungry for breakfast and I can't figure out why I'm gaining so much weight."

My mother simply refused to notice that she grossly overate while she cooked, and as a result she gained weight, eating herself to a tragic diagnosis without the faintest idea that she was harming her body by what she was eating. No one, not a doctor or a friend, told her how destructive her eating patterns were, and she was simply following in her own mother's footsteps. It was a pattern of learned behavior—her mother ate fried chicken, so did she and so did we, since it tasted so darn good.

When I considered the above, it was not surprising that specific weaknesses were passed down through my mom's side of the family. Our poor, overworked pancreases were finished before we even got started. I call that learned ignorance.

"We just love our French fries and bread," a family declares while they stuff their faces with the worst kind of nonfood.

We love our French fries and bread because everyone in our families sat around and ate them at the dinner table over good conversation and a few laughs. It was part of the family culture and training, as we were all taught to eat and drink in the same way. And so we usually got sick and died in the same way as well.

My brother and I had the same cravings as my mother and grandmother. Was this a surprise? It was not only hard on our pancreases, but all that cooked protein had created an overabundance of uric acid, which helped trash our kidneys. Then, over the years, accumulated toxins and kidney stones created blockages until our kidneys were no longer functioning properly, leaving us with frequent backaches, stiffness, and other symptoms. This was the family history, and each generation got weaker and more deficient. Grandma had glandular and organ weaknesses from poor dietary choices, which were passed down to my mother and finally to us. What a legacy!

Kelly's Story

Just as my family passed down the specific patterns and habits that created blood sugar problems, my clients had been affected by their own family patterns. For example, I met Kelly Rowan, one of the stars on the popular television series *The O.C.*, about fourteen years ago. Shortly after we met that day, she began losing her focus as her hands suddenly started to shake violently and she turned white. I could see that she was about to pass out, but before I could move forward to help, she darted out of the room. She came back a few minutes later, eating some kind of sugary treat. She was heading rapidly down the path toward diabetes and she was exhausted and scared, with no idea what to do.

An adorable girl, she was a little bit puffy, and she worked out like a maniac to keep her weight under control, counting every calorie and worrying about every morsel that passed her lips. Of course, when I looked back at her eating history, she *should* have been worried—not about her weight, but about what she was doing to herself at each "nonmeal."

Kelly grew up in Canada, where her parents smoked, drank alcohol, and ate like the rest of us did. She loved SpaghettiOs and bologna sandwiches on Wonder bread (who didn't?!), and her family dinners consisted of meat, potatoes, and a canned vegetable. She ate a typical breakfast of toast, jelly, and cereal, she snacked on peanut butter and jelly sandwiches and individually wrapped American cheese slices, and she loved going to the candy store to stock up on Gummi Bears, candy necklaces, and multicolored lollipops. At age seventeen, she started her day with coffee and a bran muffin, and she was out the door to school. She rarely, if ever, drank water (who did?), favoring pasteurized orange juice, Coke, and Tab.

As an adult, Kelly ate pasta and drank wine at least four nights a week. She had bagels or muffins for breakfast and had to have her two or three cappuccino lattes every day. Constantly exhausted, she couldn't function without her regular caffeine hits, and by the time she was twenty-one, she was so depleted, she went to her doctor for a checkup.

Because her exhaustion level was so profound, she was sure she had mononucleosis, but she didn't. After reviewing her blood tests, her doctor sent her away with a clean bill of health, but she was too exhausted and weak to care.

I told her that if she didn't radically change her eating habits, she would become an insulin-dependent diabetic, struggling with multiple symptoms for the rest of her life. I offered to help her turn her health around, and she accepted with gratitude.

Kelly was a very willing client who jumped right in and cut everything out of her diet that was processed, packaged, sugar-filled, or made with any kind of flour. She quit eating pasta, pizza, bread, all forms of sugar, and all fruit for two years. The worst part was giving up her lattes, but she did it because she was determined to get well.

I put Kelly on regular cleanses and fasts, and she used her own colema board regularly. I remember her calling me one day when she was in the middle of a seven-day fast. She felt horrible and she was not happy. I told her that her toxins were making her feel lousy and she needed to get right back on her colema board and flush her intestines. An hour later, she called me, amazed that during the colema she had passed what looked like the side of her brain. She couldn't imagine how long this toxic glob had been stuck inside her intestines, and as it flushed out, she started to sob, letting go of years of held-in emotions. Kelly was thrilled and said that she had never felt that good. Oh, the miracle of a good cleanse!

Fourteen years later, Kelly's body has changed profoundly. Her blood sugars are stable, she naturally maintains a perfect weight, and it never occurs to her to worry about it now that she understands that calorie counting is meaningless. Kelly actually eats more now than she ever did, including lots of raw fats to maintain her health and energy, and she never gains extra pounds. She exercises because she enjoys it, not because she has to, her menstrual cycle has become more balanced, and her energy is good.

Appreciative that she has lost her cravings for junk food, she feels energized and well nourished, and she says that her body looks and feels better than it did when she was twenty-five. Kelly's skin has become beautiful with very few wrinkles, so this way of eating certainly seems to be an answer to the antiaging craze. Eat what Mother Nature intended and your skin will reward you.

Kelly thinks she would have been in big trouble if she hadn't changed her eating and drinking habits. Because of her rigorous work schedule with late nights on the set, she knows that her old patterns of eating and drinking would have been her downfall. Today Kelly is calm and centered, and almost every day her energy is fantastic and she is happy and balanced.

She watches with frustration as so many of her fellow actresses fight for the perfect body. "In America, "Kelly says," "women are supposed to look a certain way. We diet and diet and we're all under so much pressure in this youth culture of ours, but the diets are too restricting and always involve deprivation. I never feel deprived anymore, and if I have a raw cookie or a piece of organic chocolate, that's great! Recently I was with some friends who were sharing a piece of heavy-duty chocolate cake. I had one bite and it was so sweet, I couldn't stand it and I was done. At that moment, I realized how much my body, my outlook, and my habits have changed. This way of eating has completely transformed my life, physically, emotionally, and mentally."

When a person eats too many refined grains or sugars that are not completely metabolized (used) in the cell, fermentation occurs, creating an anaerobic environment, forcing the oxygen out. And when there is a lack of oxygen, it enables cancer to grow. Always remember, highly refined sugars and cooked meats contribute to creating an acidic environment, which forces oxygen out, leaving behind it an unbalanced environment, a virtual breeding ground for cancer and most other kinds of diseases.

It's all in the family albums. If you write down your favorite family meals, you can start unraveling the great mystery of your own so-called diseases. It really isn't so much a health disease as it is a disease of the family fork and mouth! In other words, our indoctrinated eating and drinking patterns keep us in prison. It's true that we are what we eat, drink, and think, so if we learn the family patterns and continue to eat the same way, we have to remember the old saying "Stupid is as stupid does." In my world, it is time to get smart and stay smart.

CHAPTER 7

The Tin Man

Heavy Metals and Inorganics

DDT, pesticides, city water, and a lifetime of junk food were only a few of many causes of my accumulation of heavy metals and inorganics. Although my health had improved dramatically since I'd begun to cleanse, my knee joints were still painful and my back was always stiff. Now that my body was slowly healing and rebalancing itself, I noticed the more subtle symptoms, and I was eager to do something about them, especially my joint pain.

I went back to Dr. Walker's book about eating raw. He discussed the concept of inorganics, toxic material, and acids getting trapped in the joints, which made sense to me. But how could I get the heavy metals and inorganics *out of* my joints? I followed Dr. Walker's advice and started drinking distilled water, which he said would help the body cleanse inorganics from the joints. I drank distilled water until it was coming out of my ears, but instinctively I knew that was not going to be enough.

Logic told me that I needed to make formulas that would open up and remove any waste or toxins still stuck in my kidneys. If I allowed them to remain there, it was almost certain that my kidneys would succumb to calculus, stones, and partial solidification. All you have to do is eat processed and junk food for many years, and then voilà! Your organs start to harden.

I asked myself, *What is solidification, calcification, and hardening, anyway?* To put it simply, if the body cannot break something down, metabolize it, utilize it, turn it into energy, or fully eliminate it, then it remains inside of you and can get stuck. Once stuck, it can create a hardening at that particular place in the body and wreak havoc.

For example, if you drop an ice cream cone on the pavement, the next day it's going to be melted and stuck wherever it was left. How can it disappear? Where can it go? If there is no rain to wash it away, it'll remain there for a long, long time. It's the same with the system. If you don't utilize and get rid of undigested food and toxins, they could stay stuck there forever and you could be in big trouble.

I started designing formulas that would slowly dissolve kidney obstructions and bladder stones. As I took the formulas and drank distilled water, I captured my urine in beakers and could actually see the sandlike sediment being eliminated. When I held it under a phase contrast microscope, I could see not only the sandy sediment, I also saw spiral-like casts that had formed on the inside of my ureter. This verified to me that my formulas were doing exactly what I wanted them to do. What a fascinating process!

Slowly, over the next few months, as my kidneys and bladder got cleansed, I noticed that my urine stream increased. The unexpected benefit was that my lower back pain and stiffness started to dissipate. During all those years that I'd experienced pain and stiffness in my lower back, it never occurred to me that it was connected to my kidneys. I was too young to have kidney problems, or so I thought, and my symptoms didn't seem to indicate it. But when I realized that I was dissolving calculus and stones, I became even more convinced that solidification was a problem throughout our bodies. It affected not only the elderly. It didn't matter how old you were.

When I considered myself and all the clients I'd seen over the years, the underlying theme was the same with each of us: too much junk food, not enough water or the right kind of water, and never a time when we gave our bodies a rest or a cleanse. We had collected a lifetime of toxins, heavy metals, poisons, additives, preservatives, pollution, and pharmaceutical drugs. What did we expect? Just because we went to the bathroom didn't mean we were getting rid of all that waste. We were all eating and drinking ourselves solid, with no idea of what was actually going on inside of our struggling systems. How could we expect normal functioning from our organs and glands when they were too solidified to work properly?

Think for a moment about a baby's supple body. At the time we are born, our joints are limber, our organs are usually clear and running at 100 percent capacity, and our tissues are soft and have good integrity. Over the years, through incorrect eating and drinking patterns, our organs, tissues, and glands become harder and harder, until we feel like the Tin Man, too rusty to move. That is how we lose our flexibility as we age.

The deterioration process goes on as the malfunctioning organ, gland, or tissue gives us a signal—a symptom. When it becomes uncomfortable enough, we try to stop that discomfort by taking a drug. But will that drug do the solidified body part any good? Of course not. It may mask the symptoms and cause the body to stop crying out for help temporarily, but it will never correct the problem. How can it possibly correct anything? All that drug can do, if it's not eliminated, is create more problems and possibly add to the solidification process.

The truth is that man-made pharmaceuticals do not detoxify the human body. Neither can a drug cleanse solidification out of the organs, tissues, and glands. From my extensive research, I have learned that the only substances capable of healing are those that come directly from the earth—the true building blocks for the body. Creation *does* cleanse and regenerate if we give nature's substances a chance to work. How long has it taken to solidify our system? Possibly a lifetime.

If we want to have a new body, *it is absolutely essential* to remove anything that is slowly shutting down the various systems of that body.

Using my herbal formulas to support the body in removing the blockages, I saw a major difference. It was beautiful to me, watching the herbs work synergistically with the body as they slowly, powerfully, and methodically supported the body until balance was restored. The body could and would completely heal, since an herb was nature's food— meant to feed us and to restore our health.

You can't beat nature's perfection.

To Salt or Not to Salt

A significant discovery on my way to restoring balance was in the consumption of salt. When I eliminated table salt altogether from my diet, my joints stopped swelling. Further research into the balance of minerals, including the importance of specific minerals and salt at the cellular level, showed me that due to the refining process, table salt was not only unbalanced—it was also detrimental to our bodies and internal systems in general. That raised a conflict, however, because we need salt to survive.

I theorized that when man took anything from nature and isolated out a single molecule, it usually would lead to major imbalances. Because anticaking agents such as aluminum are used in the salt refining process, a consistent diet of such table salt could lead to an overload of this potentially harmful heavy metal. Please be aware that some recent researchers are finding links between aluminum accumulation and Alzheimer's.

Furthermore, during the refining of table salt, the macro- and microminerals, the elementals, and the isotopes are mostly removed, and the sodium chloride molecule is isolated from its elemental friends. When a sodium chloride molecule tries standing on its own without the other elements found in unrefined salt, the body treats the lone sodium chloride molecule as a toxic element. Therefore, on its own, coupled with the way that the food industry presents it, table salt is largely an unbalanced element.

As a result, our poor bodies have grown accustomed to regarding table salt as a toxin, forcing it out of the cells, as we become swollen and dehydrated when we eat too much table salt. When the isolated sodium chloride molecule is forced out of the cell, it gets pushed out in a water solution that surrounds the cells, creating an interrupt in the electrical interaction between cells. As the water and the sodium chloride molecules get pushed out of the cells, they become dehydrated—the reason our body gets thirsty. Who doesn't crave a gallon of water after eating Chinese food with all that soy sauce?

In my estimation, it seems that table salt could create an imbalance in the relationship between sodium and potassium, which has everything to do with the production of our cellular energy. We need to understand, however, that a salt-free diet is dangerous to our health. Unrefined sea salt is essential for our survival. If properly balanced, unrefined sea salt-salt is one effective way to keep water inside the system, helping keep bodily fluids and the pH in balance while it helps prevent us from becoming too acidic. Salt is also a vitally important component of bone. If your salt levels are too low, you can suffer from depression, hormonal imbalances, and even cancer.

In my experience, the better the quality of the salt along with proper hydration, the more significant the changes in overall health. It is easy to get confused by so many different salts on the market, but as usual, the purest unrefined sea salts have had the most balanced effects on my health and on the health of my clients.

Mineral Thieves

While I was researching salts, I was making herbal formulas for my stiff joints. Since I was still juicing, drinking distilled water, and taking my herbal formulas, I was making headway with my joint pain and stiffness. As I removed years of inorganics and waste from my joints, I started to regain flexibility and feel less like an arthritic old man. In fact, I was starting to feel vibrant, recapturing my ability to move with freedom. I was loving life.

I recorded my new findings until one day I wondered if our bodies were getting enough minerals from our food. If these elements need to be replaced every day to keep our bodily fluids in balance and our organs, glands, tissues, and bones fed, from where are we getting the correct minerals in the correct and balanced form to accomplish this?

The answer I found out is that we're stealing them!

It's true. We are unconscious mineral thieves, stealing needed minerals directly from our own bones because of our diets of processed sugar, flour, soda, etc. These kinds of junk foods create such a high degree of acidity, we need a tremendous amount of minerals to keep the bodily fluids in balance. Because we're not getting adequate amounts of minerals from our food, the body is forced to steal it from our bones. It's like a slow, silent robbery is being perpetrated against us, by us. As we steal these minerals, we weaken our bone structure and we eventually start to break apart. No wonder there's so much osteoporosis in this country!

Americans consume more milk and dairy products than most other places in the world, so why are the numbers of people with osteoporosis skyrocketing? Think about it. We drink pasteurized milk until it is coming out of our ears, and still our bones are brittle and our body fluids are out of balance. And we think we're doing a great thing when we drink milk. We tell ourselves we're getting calcium, which builds strong bones. In fact, many of us thought for the longest time (some of us still do) that we were adequately replenishing our minerals with one big glass of cold milk.

How many times have we been given this kind of misinformation? The truth is that the calcium in milk that helps build bones and keep our body fluids in balance cannot do it alone. As I stated before, all the minerals and elements working together as a team are vital to our good health. Calcium alone is not enough, especially when we consider the damaging effects of pasteurized and homogenized dairy, as previously discussed.

When the body steals minerals from its own bones, by the way, it is not only stealing calcium. It tries to steal whatever minerals it needs. As a result, our already deficient bodies are forced, in a sense, to cannibalize our own mineral-deficient bones to stabilize the severely out-of-balance bodily fluids. By the time the body is forced to do just that, we have been silently struggling and out of balance for years. Therefore, when we sit down to a huge glass of milk and a ton of cooked-to-death food, our bodies wonder what we expect them to do with all this stuff.

Dr. Walker insists that the cooking process changes and denatures most food particles. This is why certain undigested food particles turn into toxic sludge and end up being deposited, along with other inorganics, into our joints, tissues, organs, and fat cells. Then we devour a sugary dessert, our bodies swings dangerously acidic, and the cycle starts all over again.

Cooking Your Food to Death

To research cooking food to death, I studied what happened to overcooked fats and proteins. My discoveries were shocking and deeply unsettling. After the cooking process, besides the destruction of precious fats and needed enzymes, the remaining fat molecules are not at all the same as they had been in their original, raw form. This cooked fat is affecting our bodies in ways that none of us could possibly imagine.

While I was studying the effects of cooking fats and proteins, the craze was high-protein, low-fat diets. Fat was definitely the bad guy, according to the so-called authorities who planted this idea in people in the first place and were working like the devil to keep it going. Do some research for yourself. How many foods can you buy at the grocery store with labels that read in big, bold letters: NO FAT or REDUCED FAT. We have been programmed to think that we're doing ourselves a favor by cutting out fat. If we eat less fat or no fat, we figure, then we won't *get* fat! But that is just not true. Just eating less fat alone will not protect you from getting fat or from developing high cholesterol or hardening of the arteries.

The correct fats, eaten in their raw form, however, *can* perform miracles. If the governmental organizations who label our foods claim to protect the public, then perhaps they should do some scientific homework to present the correct information. I question from where they are getting their scientific data, because Creation doesn't change its rules.

Since we can't argue with facts, let's look back for a minute. In the early 1900s, statistics reveal that about one in a thousand people suffered from heart disease. In the early 1940s, due to the processing of foods, at least half of us started developing some form of heart disease. Today, one of every two people develops some form of heart disease and dies from it. The fast-food industry overprocesses and overcooks our meats, including their fats, which has taken a tragic toll on our bodies.

The most important thing about fat or protein is that the correct form enters the body, which is raw and uncooked—the way it came from Mother Nature. It needs to stay in its original form, untouched, uncooked, unaltered, and unprocessed, because the body looks at any other form as a foreign invader.

When a fat gets cooked for as little as three minutes at a relatively low temperature, it not only kills the inherent enzyme in that food that is so vital in breaking down and delivering the fat, it also flips the hydrogen bonds into something new, called a trans fat. Now the biochemistry has been radically changed for the worse, since a trans fat molecule is unstable and can't be broken down properly.

One of the damaging properties of trans fat is how it can get stuck on the inside of the artery walls, becoming arterial plaque. To give an analogy, the molecules of cooked fat solidify like a piece of soft, mushy bubble gum. The more the trans fat gets stuck to the arterial walls, the more likely we will develop blockages throughout the entire arterial system. This makes the artery too clogged, and the more narrow it becomes, the more likely it is that high stress or poor dietary habits will encourage this mushy bubble gum or plaque to break off.

If this happens, even temporarily, in any one of the arteries that supply blood to the heart, an interruption occurs in the electric current going to the heart, which can trigger a heart attack. Most fast-food places are cooking with hydrogenated oils that have already been turned into trans fats. It seems like a miracle to me that my friends and I are still standing. How did our arterial systems look by the time we were eighteen years old? I shudder to think! In fact, doctors are shocked to see advanced arteriosclerosis in too many children these days. As usual, we are doing this to ourselves.

The solution is simple:

Stop eating junk!

Is that a mystery to the medical establishment? They have supposedly been looking for a cure for heart disease all these years, and yet the statistics of people suffering heart attacks in this country are abysmal. When you look for a cure, don't you first need to look for the cause? They use the same meaningless slogan, "We are looking for a cure." What about the obvious indicators of possible causes that we've known about for years? Why hasn't any of this information become public knowledge?

Let's face it. If big business were really interested in correcting the health of this nation, they would teach the public about the causes, as I'm doing in this book. But they are not!

That means *we* have to wake up to the fact that our only protection lies in educating *ourselves* about our own bodies and what we are putting into them. We are the cause, and we are the cure. Our only real insurance policy is ourselves.

Cooked vs. Raw, Live vs. Dead

Imagine if every school-age child knew that he or she should eat only foods that came directly from the ground, land, or sea, untouched, unchanged, and unaltered. This is the only real food designed by Creation for the human body. Based on my clinical practice, it is my opinion that if we all ate real food, the health of this nation would radically change for the good and diseases would disappear rapidly.

But unfortunately, we feed our kids garbage, and then we send them off to school for more garbage. When they get sick, we give them a toxic drug that can't possibly remove the cause because we are the cause in the first place. Most drugs don't cure anything, and once again, we are in the same vicious cycle. We feed our kids junk food, their bodies get clogged with toxins and hydrogenated oils, and we just keep sending little Jimmy back to school with lunch money. We need to change this cycle of ignorance and take responsibility for what we are creating.

Because of this frightening state of affairs, I continue to make sure that my clients stay away from hydrogenated oils, as I include a broad range of raw fats in their diets. Fats and oils in their raw form can help to emulsify and slowly remove the hardened trans fats that are stuck to the arterial walls. But what about cooked proteins? The doctors tell us to cook meat well, and I know a lot of people who prefer steak well done.

The facts are that cooking an animal protein too long at a high temperature kills the protease, the enzyme in protein that breaks down the meat into individual amino acids. Protease acts like a mailman for each individual amino acid, the building blocks of protein. How do you expect to get your mail (the amino acids, the building blocks for your body) if you kill the mailman (the enzyme)? No mailman, no mail delivery. It's the same with animal proteins. The more you cook the meat, the more concentrated and tough it becomes, making it more difficult to break down and release the individual amino acids.

When these amino acids are not fully broken down, chunks of undigested protein can create an excess of uric acid, acidifying the system even further. The more acidic our bodies become, the more the oxygen is forced out, and the easier it is for cancer and viruses to proliferate. At the same time, parasites absolutely love it when the improper digestion of protein happens, as they also thrive in a low-oxygen environment. Parasites live off undigested protein.

The body will always continue its valiant attempt to digest this undigested protein. The body never gives up trying to restore balance, its main objective at all times. But this means that we have to use, or steal, more of our own precious enzymes to break down the protein, and our bodies suffer greatly. This led me to research the specific things we were constantly consuming that would cause the body to respond negatively. This powerful information would expose the real culprits that were creating imbalances and other problems in our bodies.

In researching our amazing immune system responses, I learned that when something enters our system that our body does not want, our body sends out its own sort of military to go after these invaders. Our great internal military are called white cells, and like the army, navy, air force, or marines, we have different branches. The white cells such as leukocytes, phagocytes, eosoinophils, neutrophils, and monocytes are the various branches of our body's internal military, each responding and mobilizing its forces depending on the type of threatening invaders. Responding to our particular needs at any given time, our body sends out the specific branch of white cells that best serves the purpose. Our system simply knows that that particular invader should not be here as it prepares to surround, destroy, and eliminate it.

Each time the body feels threatened, it mobilizes its forces and the white cell count rises. I was shocked to discover that our white cell count rises dramatically in response to cooked food, our body recognizing it as a foreign invader, a toxin, or a poison.

The tradition of incorrect eating has become a normal part of our lifestyle, as it unnaturally forces the body to fight the cooking process by constantly digging deep into its reserve energy. This is why so many people are walking around tired all the time, especially after a big meal. We are paying an extremely high energy price, as we cause our limited metabolic enzyme banks as well as our digestive enzyme banks to unnecessarily mobilize every time we eat cooked food. As we do this, we are rapidly deteriorating our bank accounts.

The faster we use up enzymes, the faster we age, and the more susceptible we become to invaders. This rapidly depletes our reserves of both enzymes that could have been used for other, more important functions, not only shortening the length of life, but greatly affecting our quality of life as well.

In medical pathology, an excessive amount of white corpuscles in the blood is referred to as leukocytosis, which was originally considered normal in 1846, because it seemed to register the same in everyone's blood. Digestive leukocytosis was considered normal until Paul

Kouchakoff, M.D., upset the theory by proving that if food was eaten raw and uncooked, the body would not produce leukocytosis. Cooking was the cause of digestive leukocytosis.

In a 1975 book called *Survival into the 21st Century*, by Viktoras Kulvinskas, M.S., he writes about Dr. Kouchakoff's studies. "Dr. Kouchakoff," Kulvinskas tells us, "divided leucocytosis into four distinct groups, according to the way these foods reacted in the blood." They are as follows:

1. A raw food produces no increase in white cells.

2. Commonly cooked foods produce leukocytosis.

3. Pressure-cooked foods produce greater leukocytosis than non-pressure-cooked foods.

4. Manufactured foods such as wine, vinegar, white sugar, and ham offend the most.

Kulvinskas goes on to say, "Prepared or processed meat (cooked, smoked, and salted) brought on the most violent reactions equivalent to the leukocytosis count manifest in poisoning." He also found that a largely raw food diet offsets the adverse effect of a small amount of cooked food so as not to cause leukocytosis.

Kulvinskas later wrote, "Cooked food has lost more than 85% of its nutrient value. It acts as a poison in the body, especially if it ingested hot, that is, warmer than 100 degrees F. Most cooked foods are eaten at a temperature of 180 degrees F. Until the temperature is reduced to that of your body, the whole metabolism is in a state of emergency. . . . Considering the small temperature range at which enzymes are active, you are doing similar harm by eating cold food. Frozen protein in the form of ice cream is putrefactive in the digestive system."

See how destructive it is to cook food? The stunner is that judging by the dates of these studies, this information has been available since the 1940s. Just think how many lives could have been saved if everyone in America had this information! I was convinced that cooked protein could be a strong contributor to cancer, since it leaves too much excess uric acid in the body, which, in turn, creates too much bodily acidity, forcing oxygen out, and setting the stage for cancer to grow.

Carol Alt's Story

About ten years ago, I got a frantic call from Carol Alt, a former super-model, who was in a major health crisis. She had just returned from film-ing *Supermodels in the Rainforest*, her abdomen was bloated, and she couldn't figure out why. Looking her best at all times was crucial for someone who made her living as a model. She also had sinus problems, and she begged to see me as soon as possible, to which I agreed.

Carol, a superbly beautiful woman, had grown up on the Standard American Diet. What else was new? She loved to eat pasta with meat-balls and sausage, as well as pancakes or French toast that her father made for the family on Sunday mornings. She also ate cereals, bagels, butter, orange and cream soda, chocolate, TV dinners and frozen veg-etables in plastic bags. She rarely, if ever, drank water. As a result, she had sinus problems, hypoglycemia, exhaustion, and what looked like systemic *Candida albicans*, an overgrowth of fungus.

As a model, Carol was forced to stay underweight for her frame. When she felt tired and listless, she took some so-called herbal drops that were supposed to give her an energy lift. Pretty soon she was using a nasal spray to unclog her perpetual runny nose, she got a recurring sinus infection, and her doctor prescribed several rounds of antibiotics. She also chewed Tums like candy, popping eight or nine before bed each night. During our first phone call, I asked her my favorite trick ques-tion—if she thought she ate healthy.

"Are you kidding?" she answered. "No! I start every day with Scotch and coffee, and I'm eating nachos as we speak! Irish coffee is my main-stay. I live on it!"

At least she wasn't lying to herself. As she filled me in on her abysmal eating habits, I heard her desperation and I decided to take her on. She was so elated that right then and there she went over to the sink and poured out what was left of her beloved Irish coffee—the last one she ever had.

During her first appointment, I gave her a solid foundation and she started implementing my suggestions that very day. She was taking Afrin, Cipro (an antibiotic), Tums, 222's (a combo of aspirin, caffeine, and codeine), and Nyquil. When I suggested that she ease off some of the drugs she was taking, she cut out everything, all at once. By the time Carol's diet was 75 percent raw, she was hungry for education and she soaked it all in, repeating my methods to herself out loud. Because she was so compliant, rapid changes took place in her body, and after only three days, her allergies and congestion were gone, her headaches had disappeared, and her fatigue was diminishing.

Over the next few months, it was a pleasure being Carol's mentor. Within the next thirty days, Carol's body morphed before our very eyes as she took control of her internal environment. Her body started to achieve balance, her *Candida albicans* started to diminish, and her severe abdominal bloating disappeared. I spent hours in my kitchen showing her how to make raw recipes and shakes, and she was in seventh heaven.

To this day, she has remained loyal to the principles I taught her in 1996. In fact, my methods influenced her so profoundly, she went on to write a book called *Eating in the Raw*, based on my eating principles.

Louie's Story

When Louie first came to me, he hobbled into my office wearing one shoe and holding the other in his hand, and he was in agony. Louie suffered from a chronic case of gout, and the minute he healed from one gout attack, the next one was waiting to strike.

As he sat in my office that afternoon, his gout-ridden toe was swollen beyond recognition, looking like a strawberry. The pain was so great he was practically incapacitated. I took one look at that toe and thought, *Here I go again!* I didn't know the first thing about gout or how to treat it, and Louie was in a major crisis. But I did know that Louie's history would give me my first clue.

Louie was five foot eight and weighed about two hundred pounds, with a gut so big he looked like a bloated Santa Claus. He suffered from acid reflux, gas, bloating, and severe constipation. His elbows and knees were almost completely locked up, and his family had a history of heart disease. In other words, Louie was a wreck. When we got to his dietary history, everything started to make sense.

Louie dearly loved meat, and the more cooked the better. He loved to barbecue the heck out of his steaks, which added to the amount of carcinogens in his system. Louie was a meat-and-potatoes guy, and he also loved eating chicken—and gobs of it. Rather than eating a normal amount of cooked food, Louie ate insane amounts of cooked meat at every meal, and he avoided fruits and vegetables as much as possible. His whole life revolved around meat and wine, as he lived to eat and then eat again, unsatisfied unless he pushed away from the table stuffed to the brim.

In his book *Survival into the 21st Century*, Viktoras Kulvinskas wrote, "Eating a steak may be more dangerous than smoking. One pound of charcoaled broiled steak has as much benzopyrene (cancer-stimulating agent) as in the smoke of 300 cigarettes." Mice fed benzopyrene developed leukemia and stomach tumors.

Since Louie couldn't get enough barbecued and smoked meats, many of his symptoms, particularly his severe lower backaches and kidney problems, pointed to protein poisoning. Even before I started working with him, I thought he probably had too many undigested protein bodies in his blood due to his circulation problems and high blood pressure. When we checked, Louie had very low HDL (good cholesterol) and very high LDL (bad or dangerous cholesterol). His doctors, concerned with a family history of blocked arteries, put him on high-blood-pressure medications and several others for his gout. Judging by his appearance, the drugs were not helping him, and I couldn't believe his doctor didn't have the sense to pull him off all of that cooked protein.

When I tested Louie's pH, his system was so acidic it frightened me. I just couldn't imagine the chaos taking place inside his body. A voracious eater, he was stuffing his face with so much cooked protein, there was no way his digestive system could keep up with the onslaught. He was always hot and perspiring, and he had an explosive kind of energy, as if his body and personality were about to boil over and explode.

I couldn't help but notice that the smell emanating from his body was putrid, which had nothing to do with his hygiene. In fact, when I first opened the door and he walked into my place, it smelled like something was rotting and burning in the hallway.

"What is that horrible smell out here?" I said out loud, closing the door behind Louie. When I turned around and walked back into my office, it reeked with the same smell. How could anyone smell so bad?

Louie had huge intestinal blockages. How could anyone expect to have a bowel movement after eating half a cooked cow? He also had horrible headaches, which didn't surprise me. The only thing that did surprise me was that he was still alive.

As with so many clients before him, the first thing I did was to radically change his diet, which I knew would be extremely hard for Louie, being such a meat junkie. Of course he was appalled when I told him he couldn't eat any meat for a while. Then I started to rehydrate and remineralize him slowly over a two-week period with my herbal mineral formulas. I had him juicing vegetables like crazy, drinking distilled water, and adding a minute amount of unrefined sea salt to his diet to guarantee his rehydration. I also had him transition to a diet of 50 percent raw foods with a lot of salads, which was very difficult for him. I knew that he had to start opening up his bowels to let out the trapped toxins, but the name of the game with Louie was slow and gentle. His body simply could not take an onslaught of acid dumping out of his toxic system too rapidly.

The crowning blow for Louie was when I told him to eat raw fish. When that didn't go over at all, I told him to eat lightly seared fish instead, that was raw in the middle. Louie hated fish, cooked or raw, but he toughed it out. He ended up being compliant because he was in such pain with his gout, desperate for change.

As he hydrated his body along with all the other things he was doing, he reported that he was urinating more than before. That was great, considering that Louie used to go a whole day without urinating. This gives you an idea of how much water he drank before he came to see me. Literally none. He never, ever drank any water during the day—until now, and now he was urinating frequently.

This was difficult, since he had to hobble to the bathroom with his gouty toe throbbing in pain, but we had no choice. Louie desperately needed to be rehydrated, and I needed to orchestrate it slowly. I didn't want his body to throw out acid and undigested protein too quickly, but as he continued to hydrate—drink water—and urinate, he started to feel less pressure in his lower back and kidney area. It seemed to me that Louie was starting to release some of the toxic buildup of protein that was overloading his compromised kidneys.

You can only imagine his annoyance when I made sure that he chewed each bite of food at least thirty to sixty times before swallowing. This drove Louie out of his mind, since he had previously taken pride that he could finish a large, well-done steak in less than ten minutes. Now he was forced to chew his food until it was liquid, quite a challenge with any food, and especially when he ate fish.

Guess what? As time went on, Louie not only became a fish lover, he also started to love sashimi—raw fish!

As Louie continued to follow my protocol, his gout pain lessened and he told me that he felt much calmer. When his doctor took his blood pressure and saw that it had dropped within normal range, what could he say? He was the one who had told Louie that he had high blood pressure in the first place and now, even though Louie was eating seaweed and unrefined sea salt, his blood pressure was back to normal. The doctor had never seen that, and of course Louie was as astonished as the doctor was, and more motivated than ever to follow my program. A short time later, Louie went off his high-blood-pressure medication completely, even though the doctor had said he would have to take it for the rest of his life. It had finally become obvious to Louie that his body had its own set of rules, not made up by man.

Over the next months, as his gout attacks started to subside, Louie was ecstatic. No doctor had been able to give him relief, and he was thrilled with what was taking place. His chronic stomach burning stopped in the first three days of his dietary change, he was feeling relatively normal, and he didn't need his acid reflux medication anymore, either. For a guy who popped a handful of Tums every five minutes, this was a miraculous change.

Louie started to walk and swim, and he was happy to report that even though he was pathetically out of shape, he didn't feel the same level of soreness he had previously when he started to exercise. He was getting his strength back, and better than that, he was no longer constipated. I guess my formulas were really working!

In the first three months, Louie effortlessly lost twenty-five pounds. His pH was turning more alkaline, the circulation in his arms and legs was greatly improving, and his headaches were gone. He loved the bowel cleanses and the liver/gallbladder flushes, which gave his body the leeway to detoxify and regenerate. At the end of a full year of Louie's working with me, he had lost fifty pounds. The best part was that he not only felt like a new man, he *was* a new man. All he had to do was provide his body with what it needed, and his body took care of the rest.

His body had healed his body. Louie was living proof of that. The drugs he had been given had not only masked his symptoms, but probably caused more problems. They simply could not affect the root causes of his condition in a positive way. It had been plain and simple to me that the guy needed to stop stuffing his face with all that highly cooked meat. He desperately had needed the proper hydration and nourishment, and with those, his body created changes that resulted in great health.

When I think back to the first time I met Louie, he had all but given up hope that he would ever feel halfway decent again. Thank goodness his body didn't believe that for a second, as it was crying out to him, "Just give me a chance. I can heal myself if you feed me correctly!"

God designed the human body to be a continual self-healing mechanism. Louie's body, no exception to the rule, underwent extraordinary changes in a relatively short period of time. In fact, his changes were so pronounced that his cardiologist was fascinated by the process I'd suggested. He said he'd never seen such a dramatic reversal in a person with such serious symptoms. He didn't understand it at all, but he told Louie that whatever he was doing, he needed to keep doing it. Here it was once again. Louie created his conditions by his lifestyle patterns, and then, when he changed his addictive behaviors, Louie ended up healing Louie.

Did Louie really have a disease? To me, a disease implies that we have no control getting rid of it, that we are at the mercy of it. We all hold the keys to great health in our hands; it is not in the hands of our doctors. We just need to find the courage to step up and change, which is what Louie did.

This is exactly what I continue to do with myself and my clients. We eat directly from nature, we get out of our own way and let our bodies do the only things they know how to do: heal and regenerate. What a privilege it has been for me to participate in and witness these remarkable recoveries. What an amazing way to learn and grow as we follow the correct path that will lead us straight back to renewed health.

CHAPTER 8

Sonya's Story

I had more clients than I could handle, but where on earth were they coming from? My phone never stopped ringing, and my message machine was always full, because I would spend two to three hours for a first appointment and one to two hours on a follow-up appointment with each person. They were used to walking in and out of their regular doctor's office in a few minutes with little more than a prescription to fill. But I needed to teach my clients all of the principles I'd figured out over the years so they could understand the *real* reasons why they were sick.

I taught them what created their imbalances and showed them how they created the cause themselves and how they could remove it. This was a tremendously ambitious undertaking and a terrifically frustrating process for me as well as overwhelming for my clients. The terrible truth is this: raised in a land of irresponsibility and lack of awareness about our health and what we threw in our bodies, we were conditioned *not* to take responsibility for our own health with the following message: These diseases just happen; they are a mystery, so you should come to us, the professionals, the experts, and we'll take care of it quickly with a pretty little colored pill.

Today, we can see from the escalation of major health problems in this country that those pretty little pills have never been, are not now, and never will be the answer to anything.

Breakthroughs

My apartment was full to the brim with herbal experiments and formulas. I refused to take chances on other people, but I would try anything on myself, to test and improve my formulas. I just started linking things and working backward to discover what caused the underlying imbalances and how to correct them.

After witnessing remarkable healings and recoveries, I knew I was on the right track. I researched the next "incurable" health problem or concocted the newest herbal formulas to help heal a long line of sick and ailing bodies, which took patience, persistence, perseverance, and experimentation. I compiled evidence based on my practice that showed me even more crucial information, including breakthrough discoveries about what was missing in our daily intake that would help create and maintain balance. I studied nutrients (in the correct forms) that should be taken daily to help maintain balance in our systems. Then I developed herbal formulas that worked in a slow, safe, and effective way and produced powerful results. Herbs were a vital key to the healing process, just as I had suspected, as they worked in a slow, safe, and powerful way to support the body in restoring health without the negative, health-destroying side effects caused by many drugs.

Over the years, the great herbalists stated clearly that herbal formulas would perform in a safer and more effective way than a drug. Now I realized why most of the herbalists were so confident. Their knowledge had been passed down over thousands of years, and they knew that for real answers and healing, we needed to look at what was being offered by Creation.

At present, an explosion of campaigns are exposing the fact that the medical and pharmaceutical industries and associated governmental agencies have systematically tried to suppress and discredit competition in the use of natural herbs and substances during the past century. Undue pressure has been placed on sick patients to "choose" traditional treatments, discouraging the pursuit of natural treatments and substances. At times patients have been forced to flee the country to obtain certain treatments or natural substances that have proven successful in the treatment of cancer and other serious diseases. At other times, important information and breakthroughs have been suppressed or discredited, and natural practitioners have been persecuted and jailed, all at the hands of a few powerful and controlling industries. It is time for these brave people and their campaigns to finally let us know that we have had very few choices and for the public to step up and put a stop to that. Education and empowerment equal freedom!

As for my own health, I was feeling terrific, and I'd never before been so healthy and strong, but every day I was inundated with calls from sick and dying people, begging me to take them on. They had serious or fairly serious health problems and had seen numerous doctors, visited many hospitals and institutions, gotten the fancy diagnoses, and taken a variety of pharmaceuticals. Now they were not only still sick, but also many were in desperate situations with nowhere to turn.

The enormous pressure was taking a toll on my body, and I needed a break because I was getting burned out. I decided to start telling my clients, the very next day, that I would be taking some time off. But if you want to make God laugh, make plans.

I awakened the day after my big decision to take some time off, ready to begin phoning my clients to break the news to them. But when I reached over to make the first call, the phone rang. I answered it. Susan, a close friend, wanted me to schedule a meeting with some desperate people, a woman named Sonya and her boyfriend, Steve.

When I told her that I just couldn't do it right now, she literally begged me to meet with them—as a favor to her. Sonya was twenty-three years old and she had been diagnosed with cervical cancer. Reluctantly, I agreed to meet with Sonya, never anticipating how she was about to throw me for a loop.

When I met Sonya and Steve, they began to tell me the facts:

Sonya, a beautiful French Canadian woman with long, gorgeous hair and a strong French accent, had seen her gynecologist, a well-respected doctor in Los Angeles. When he told her she had a serious problem—cervical cancer—Sonya was shocked, unable to imagine how this could happen to her. She also was informed that she needed a radical hysterectomy as well as the removal of some of her lymph nodes.

Needless to say, she was terrified, shocked, and depressed. She always had wanted children, and both she and Steve were in disbelief. Sonya not only wanted to live; she also wanted to have a child someday. Maybe another doctor would have a different opinion and offer an easier, milder healing possibility that was effective but not so dangerous and radical.

Steve arranged a meeting with a reputable doctor at a well-respected cancer institution, but the new doctor agreed that Sonya needed a radical hysterectomy and the removal of some of her lymph nodes—right away. Once back in California, they decided to go for a third opinion, to a top oncologist. While Sonya was waiting for results, her original gynecologist was so furious that she had the audacity to seek other opinions, she pressured Sonya into having a biopsy to confirm her diagnosis. "You need a radical hysterectomy and a removal of some of your lymph nodes," said the doctor, agreeing with all the rest.

When they finished their story, I told them that if they wanted to go outside the medical system, it would be a massive undertaking. Over a four-hour period, I explained, as best I could, that the intensity of the needed protocol to possibly reverse her cancer would be a massive challenge for everyone. "Everyone who knows and loves you," I warned her, "will think you're insane for even attempting it. If you cross the line and choose to try something alternative, the amount of criticism and lack of agreement you'll be facing are going to be insane." I needed to prepare them both for imminent emotional battering.

Sonya and Steve needed to fully understand the stress and pressure that would come from family, friends, and the medical community as they went against their doctors' suggestions. It was the same old problem. We all were conditioned to believe that traditional cancer treatments were the only safe procedure, even though many people who went that route ended up dead. While the medical community swore that the patient had died from the cancer, I believed most of them died from complications resulting from the barbaric treatments. In my opinion, these treatments only set the stage for cancer to return with a vengeance, which it usually did.

Sonya's poor lifestyle choices had created the environment in which cancer could grow inside of her. She would have to completely change her ways. But understanding this and actually making the herculean effort to take back control of a toxic and cancerous environment were two completely different things. I could advise Sonya to eat and drink what I considered to be the healthiest choices. I could make her numerous powerful herbal formulas, and even if she were 100 percent compliant, I still didn't know if she had enough metabolic reserve to win this battle. What about her emotional and psychological states? Was she up to the task? Did she have enough will to fight back? Could she get past all of her fear from her doctors' dismal diagnosis, and did she have the strength to really go for it? Could she withstand other people's fear systems that might be constantly breaking down her belief that this treatment was the way to go?

Sonya's eating and drinking patterns were abysmal right from the start. You probably won't be surprised to learn that she always had been a milk freak. For breakfast, she ate commercial cereal with pasteurized milk, and she drank more milk throughout the day with croissants, pastries, toast, and jelly. She gorged on white bread and peanut butter and jelly sandwiches, which she washed down with—you guessed it—a great big glass of milk. At school, she ate sugary pastries with her cafeteria food. Her after-school snacks were canned and powdered soups, with nary a fresh vegetable crossing her lips. She devoured cookies, chips, Jell-O, or cake, and every once in a while she ate fruit, but she didn't really like it because, as she put it, "It just wasn't very exciting."

Dinners were strictly meat and potatoes, with canned or microwaved vegetables. Sonya never had been served a vegetable that wasn't totally mushy, and she told me that her father once cooked the Thanksgiving turkey in the microwave! After dinner, she ate ice cream and pie because she always had been thin. She could eat whatever she wanted, and she got away with it—or so she thought.

Sonya drank sodas when she wasn't drinking milk or concentrated and processed juices. She rarely drank a glass of plain water, preferring Tang or Nestlé's Quik. She took her coffee loaded with sugar, and she had another favorite: regular full-salt V8 juice. She thought it was healthy because there were pictures of vegetables on the can of V8, but it was loaded with refined salt. In fact, her entire diet was a barrage of sugar and junk, creating fermentation and forcing oxygen out at the cellular level—the perfect environment for cancer to grow.

Only bad eating, drinking, and lifestyle patterns can create a toxic, alien internal bodily environment in the first place.

I realized that my clients' successes came from all the factors I had linked over many years of work. I now could determine what factors caused the body to weaken and how to pull it back by changing what people ate and drank. If they did the work, I knew the kind of herbal formulas that could help rebalance the body, but a patient's compliance was another thing altogether. Taking control of this imbalanced and out-of-control environment would be a monumental undertaking for Sonya.

Drugging the Symptoms

There had been signs and symptoms of Sonya's crisis all along the way that everyone had ignored. Her doctors had been prescribing drugs for vaginal infections and discharges since she was a teenager. Had anyone ever stopped to wonder why she was having problems in the first place? Symptoms of imbalance were right under her doctors' noses, but they didn't look for the cause because they were never taught to remove the cause. Instead, they drugged the symptoms, hoping the condition would magically disappear. Since symptoms are the body's signals for help, if you shove them down with a drug, your internal environment continues its descent into hell.

Remember: a symptom can never disappear if you don't remove the original cause.

For a doctor to declare Sonya cancer-free, I explained, we had to change the internal environment so profoundly that the tissue level eventually changed, which could take a while. Once the tissue in which the cancer was thriving became healthy and oxygenated, when the internal environment was right and balanced, the cancer could not live. But I had no way to know how long it would take.

"What kind of guarantee can you give me that Sonya is going to be okay?" Steve asked. Steve's question was absurd, but cancer is a terrible thing to have to grasp, especially after so many doctors wanted to pick Sonya's body apart, piece by piece.

"There's no way I can give you a guarantee," I said. "But if you want to go with her doctors' advice that she needs a radical hysterectomy and the removal of some of her lymph nodes, be my guest!"

"Will you work with us?" Steve asked me. The dread rose up my spine. I knew what I was getting myself into, but I agreed to help. Sonya, Steve, and I all had been conditioned by a system that insisted a sick person should hand all power of choice over to "them" and do exactly as he or she was told—whether or not it made sense. We were about to do something different. My mind scattered for a few moments as I struggled to figure out where to start. Sonya decided to call her doctor and tell him that she wasn't having the surgery done. Her doctor wrote back a letter admonishing her for taking unnecessary risks with her life.

Undaunted by her doctor's tactics, I immediately took Sonya off all foods that were contributing to her problems. "We have to do some very radical things," I kept reminding her, "that will most likely freak out your friends and family."

We were fortunate that Sonya's boss was willing to give her time off. I focused on the top priority—to rapidly remove the massive amount of toxins that were buried and layered in Sonya's large and small intestines, liver, gallbladder, and kidneys. I needed to open up all these elimination channels simultaneously to neutralize the problem quickly. At the moment, the toxins in her system were contributing to turning her body extremely acid, forcing oxygen out, giving the cancer a perfect environment for growth.

On the first day, along with taking my detoxifying formula multiple times, Sonya took other herbal intestinal cleanses and did colemas twice that day. She was dumping so many toxins and acids, they were burning and blistering her sphincter on the way out. By the next day she had a raging fever, since the toxins were being pulled into her blood so rapidly, her body was automatically mobilizing mass defense forces to deal with them. Sonya's temperature rose so high at one point that I told Steve to pack her in cold towels. I'd been prepared for something like this, but Sonya's reaction was much more severe than Kathy's.

Sonya was busy with my protocols all day long, and Steve and I supported her as she took several of my detoxifying formulas, all at the same time. I shifted her protocol according to what her body was telling me through its biochemical fluctuations, the purpose being to alkalize her system until balance was regained. This is just one very small part of the picture.

Steve protected Sonya from outside pressure while her doctors, family, and friends, their fears well implanted by the medical and pharmaceutical industries, began to exert pressure on him, just as I'd warned. They called what she was doing "crazy and risky" (as if what they were suggesting was safe and sound!), pushing hard for her to go back to her regular doctor before she got herself into "more trouble."

I was back in the pressure cooker as people kept telling me I had to be careful that Sonya's doctors didn't sue me. Everything I was doing was completely legal, since I was following the rules of Mother Nature. Big business didn't like us, and they made sure we felt the pressure of bucking a system that was already set in place. The things I was having Sonya do did not coincide with the existing medical system's traditional cancer treatments.

Sonya was now dumping strings of tirelike material out of her intestines—the toxins and mucus that had been clogging her system for a lifetime. Her life became greatly simplified. It was all about going to the bathroom to the kitchen to the bedroom and back to the bathroom again. Sonya was clearing out years of toxins that were blocking her liver and gallbladder, and these organs needed to be softened so they could do their job. If the liver, one of the body's major organs of detoxification, is not operating at full capacity, the toxins will not be filtered out and fully eliminated. Instead they keep recirculating in the blood, and Sonya could not allow that to happen. Since the liver also is responsible for metabolizing hormones, they would remain seriously out of balance unless we cleansed and regenerated that organ.

I knew that the liver, with the pancreas and the adrenals, helped to control and balance the blood sugars, which helped to control the amount of oxygen inside every cell. An imbalance inside the cells could create a low-oxygen or anaerobic environment. Since cancer flourishes in an anaerobic environment, balancing the blood sugar would help to control the body's overall health.

As I started Sonya on a process of slowly softening and cleaning out her liver and gallbladder, she was so toxic, I couldn't depend on a traditional liver/gallbladder flush. I was back to the drawing board, creating and combining formulas to clear the way through her toxic and overloaded liver and gallbladder while regenerating and rebuilding them. I had her on many different formulas simultaneously that worked on her intestines, her liver and gallbladder, pancreas, spleen, thymus, kidneys and bladder, blood, uterus, ovaries, cervix, and her entire hormonal system.

Sonya drank fresh juices and water throughout each day, slowly rehydrating herself while I helped to remineralize her with herbal formulas and foods. With the addition of enzyme therapy, she was waging a tough battle to see how fast she could remove a lifetime of toxins and poisons, the results of a diet not meant for human consumption. It had taken approximately twenty-three years for her body to fall apart. She had been gambling with her youth, and she was losing.

Remember this: *No one can get away with eating and drinking anything they want just because it tastes good and they are young.*

Sonya was juicing constantly while transitioning her diet from processed and junk food to a healthy combination of both cooked and raw foods. We were slowly removing all that had blocked and hardened her organs, glands, and other bodily systems while she was feeding her blood with what I believed had been missing all these years. The trouble was that there was no way she could eat the huge variety of foods daily that would fill in the gaps. I needed to create herbal formulas that would nourish and rebalance her blood.

Over the next few months, we had to get *into* Sonya's body the nutrients (building blocks) she'd been missing for a lifetime. If and when we could finally feed those nutrients into her system, Sonya's tissues, her organs, her glands, and her blood could correct themselves and give her body a fighting chance to turn around her condition. But these specific nutrients had to be in perfect balance and easy to assimilate, in order not to tax her body and subsequently force it to use its metabolic reserve to digest. I needed to protect her energy and feed her at the same time, so I looked to herbs as well as other foods made by Creation. There was nothing more important than to feed Sonya's body with herbs, living food rich with enzymes, and living electrical nutrients for her electrical body. She ate as I instructed, she took a myriad of my herbal formulas, and I could tell she was definitely making progress.

I eventually changed her protocols to accommodate the radical changes taking place in her healing body, tuning every system like I was sitting in front of a huge control panel, subtly working each intricate button. The slightest adjustment was crucial for all the systems to work synergistically, a daily balancing act. But as we balanced her blood and body fluids, tissues, organs, and glands, the healing dance of Sonya's body was being performed before our very eyes. What a miracle to observe!

We worked together every day for four months, with Sonya's body going through both subtle and radical changes at the same time. Steve was absorbing the brunt of the pressure from their fear-based family and friends as they tried to twist his arm to bring her back to a doctor for a biopsy. His indoctrination as well as outside pressure were getting the better of him, while we were bucking the system, going against the grain of conventional medicine. Steve knew that Sonya's doctors offered no hope or solutions to return her to health. But common opinion was that if you had cancer, you went to your doctor for testing, and possible mutilation and poisoning.

Eventually, unbeknownst to me, Steve and Sonya succumbed to the pressure by going back to the third-opinion oncologist for a biopsy. This was a little over four months after we had begun, but they felt that they *had* to see what was happening, and they told me nothing about this doctor's visit.

Two weeks into the fifth month, Susan called to say that Steve and Sonya wanted to have a meeting with me and a group of her coworkers at the office where she worked before her diagnosis. I was leery, and when I walked in and saw everyone was gathered around, I felt like I was in the hot seat, as all eyes were turned toward me.

I looked at Sonya, whose eyes were welling up. "Timothy, I have something to tell you," she said. "I went back to my oncologist and got tested."

My heart dropped into my stomach

I feared that her doctor would talk her into surgery, and then chemotherapy and radiation, imagining that out of ignorance and fear, she would agree to all of it. It had taken months to get where we were, and it felt like we were about to cross the finish line after a million-mile marathon, but the race was called off at the last leg. What a hideous shame it would be to quit too soon.

The room had become ghostly quiet when Sonya turned to me, tears spilling down her cheeks, and said, "My cancer is gone. *Completely gone.* They can't find a trace of it!" A smile broke through her sobs of joy as the room exploded with congratulations. I exhaled, flooded with relief that her body had been young enough to rally so quickly. All the factors must have been right.

I must say here that even though I have described some cases of cancer that reversed naturally, please understand: not every one of my clients with cancer has survived. There were some who sustained such damaging effects from chemotherapy and radiation, even their doctors had given up on them. I could only help them buy more time and improve the quality of their last days. In fact, some patients who came to me were in such advanced stages that no one could do anything for them. With a cancer diagnosis, whether you approach it traditionally or alternatively, turning it around is the hardest work I've ever done.

We need to remember: *balance and prevention are everything.* Nothing else is more important.

The medical profession, the doctors, and the pharmaceuticals are not the cure. Their results with cancer are dismal at best, and if you survive their treatments, it's a tribute to the strength of your body to overcome adversity.

By the way, Sonya not only healed completely, but also, seven years after serious cancer, she would go on to have a healthy daughter who has recently turned three years old—yet another reminder that when we follow the laws of nature, our bodies can untangle the mess and bring about complete healing and balance.

CHAPTER 9

Water, the River of Life

One of the most important factors for survival and true life at the cellular level is water. For optimal health and balance, we must be completely hydrated at all times. In fact, I believe pure water and the living, active elements contained within it to be our greatest natural resources, the main factors that control our overall health.

I was a firsthand witness to this as I saw my health and the health of Carlos dramatically change when we properly hydrated our bodies. I recalled the huge amount of sodas and pasteurized juices Carlos had consumed, and remembered the gallons of tap water I guzzled. In fact, from the time we got up in the morning until we went to bed at night, our "drink diet" mainly consisted of canned or bottled juices with extra sugars or sweeteners, coffee, sodas, or diet sodas, with artificial sweeteners, along with pasteurized milk or caffeinated teas. Pure water rarely passed our lips, and our thirst was never satisfied because most of those beverages were actually forcing water out of our already dehydrated cells. And tap water was filled with toxic chemicals.

Sadly, sodas, juices, and poorly structured waters were only half the problem. The caffeine that everyone was consuming was not only forcing water out of the cells, but also, over time, it tired out the organs and glands.

What happens if you drink coffee, caffeinated tea, or colas? Dr. F. Batmanghelidj, author of the 1995 book *Your Body's Many Cries for Water*, had this to report:

"You are not sick, you are thirsty! Don't treat thirst with medications. . . . Chronic cellular dehydration painfully and prematurely kills. Its initial outward manifestations have until now been labeled as diseases of unknown origin. . . . Tea, coffee, or colas in place of water . . . are central nervous system stimulants: at the same time, they are dehydrating agents because of their strong diuretic action on the kidneys. One cup of coffee contains about 85 milligrams of caffeine, and one cup of tea contains 50 milligrams of caffeine. Cola drinks contain about 50 milligrams of caffeine. . . . The effect of caffeine may at times be considered desirable, but constant substituting of caffeine-containing drinks for water will deprive the body of its full capacity for the formation of hydroelectric energy. Excess caffeine will also deplete the ATP-stored energy in the brain and the body—a possible contributing factor for shorter attention span in the younger, cola-consuming generation, or chronic fatigue syndrome as a result of excess coffee consumption in later life. Excess caffeine intake will eventually exhaust the heart muscle because of its overstimulation. . . . Recently, in some experimental models, it has been shown that caffeine inhibits a most important enzyme system—PDE (phos-pho-di-esterease)—that is involved in the process of learning and development."

In my opinion, all these so-called drinks are also irritants as they whip up, overburden, and overstimulate the organs and glands. This kind of constant overworking forces our organs and glands into a continual cycle of craving these drinks to get energy going. Over the years, my clients who consumed these kinds of drinks were always fatigued as a result of this constant battering of their entire system.

Dr. Batmanghelidj found that chronic dehydration can lead to the following conditions: hypertension, ulcers, headaches, dyspeptic pain, colitis, false appendicitis pain, hiatal hernia, rheumatoid arthritis pain, lower back and neck pain, angina pain, stress and depression, high blood pressure, high cholesterol, excess body weight, overeating, asthma and allergies, sleep disorders, fatigue, and pain.

As I followed the miracle of rehydration, I watched in awe as various symptoms disappeared in many of my patients, merely by drinking the correct kind of water in the proper amounts. I became convinced about how dependent our bodies are on water.

This doctor's powerful statements were based on his clinical practice, in which he primarily used water to treat a multitude of diseases. Most of our blood, our body fluids, the majority of our organs, and our tissues are made up of water. As I stated previously, almost three quarters of the earth is covered with water, making the survival of life on our planet completely dependent on the quality of our water. Similarly, our bodies are made up of approximately 70 to 75 percent water, which means that we were created with structures almost identical, making our bodies a replication of the earth.

In the 2005 book *The Hidden Messages in Water*, Masaru Emoto writes: "We start out our life being 99 percent water, as fetuses. When we are born, we are 90 percent water, and by the time we reach adulthood we are down to 70 percent. If we die of old age, we will probably be about 50 percent water. In other words, throughout our lives we exist mostly as water."

The condition or state of the circulating fluids in our bodies is a main factor in determining our overall health, which is completely dependent on the quality and the amount of water we feed it daily. In fact, each biochemical reaction inside our bodies is totally dependent on the quality, structure, and amount of water that our cells, tissues, and organs constantly receive.

My friend Kristin is a prime example of someone who suffered from chronic dehydration with irregular heartbeats and left-arm pain for ten years. An acupuncturist by profession, she'd gone to other professionals, spent hundreds of dollars on tests with her cardiologist, and taken countless natural herbal formulas, vitamins, and minerals to rid herself of these scary symptoms. Still, she suffered greatly.

Like so many of my other clients, Kristin had tried many different things to no avail, and she'd given up hope that her symptoms would disappear. She lived with them as best she could, restricting her exercise and avoiding going up too many stairs for fear of having a heart attack. In her midforties, she was not overweight, but she lived every day in fear. She knew enough to be aware that her skipped heartbeats and

left-arm pain were indications of something, but so far no one had figured out specifically what.

Having heard of my herbal formulas and anticipating an appropriate
heart formula, Kristin was eager to start my protocols as soon as possible. But after asking her a few questions, I knew exactly what she had to
do. Very simply, she needed to drink water because she *never* drank any
unless she was dying of thirst.

When I told her that she needed to rehydrate her body by drinking
adequate amounts of the right kind of water every day (explained, in
detail, later in the book), she still didn't get it. "Okay," she said, "I'll
drink more water, but what about the formulas for my heart?"

"In my opinion," I told her, "you need nothing but water—pure,
structured, and balanced water."

"Okay," she said. "I'll drink water. I promise. But when do I get my
heart formulas?"

I tried again. "You don't need formulas," I repeated. "You don't
need anything right now but water."

Sometimes it takes a little time for these concepts to sink in, and I
could tell Kristin thought I was out of my mind. She said, "You've got to
be kidding me! You mean to tell me that I've seen everyone in Los
Angeles to help correct my skipped heartbeats and all you can tell me is
to drink water?"

I told her yes.

She left that day, determined to rehydrate her system, but she still
didn't believe that by simply drinking water, she could turn her
situation around. Some weeks later, however, she called me with
miraculous news. She had followed my advice and her skipped heartbeats were gone! This was the first time in ten years that she'd been
symptom-free.

"I can't believe it!" she said. "All I ever needed was to drink the right
amount and the right kind of water [explained later]. Wow, if I'd known
that, I could have saved myself countless hours of anguish and tons of
money. Thank God I did what you told me to do!"

What Chronic Dehydration Can Do

1. Every organ in the body can function only according to the level
   at which it is hydrated, meaning we have only as much energy as
   the level of bodily hydration.

2. Dehydration can greatly compromise your digestive process. You need water to help your body make enzymes, and to act as the mailmen to carry them wherever they need to go. At least 50 percent of my clients' cases of constipation were caused by dehydration.

3. We need water to eliminate toxins from the body through the skin, the bowels, the kidneys, and the bladder. A dehydrated body has a difficult time eliminating these toxins. *The solution to pollution is dilution.*

4. All messages in the body are sent from the brain in electrical currents. Water is the carrier of the conduits for that electricity.

5. All nutrients for the body can be delivered to the cell only in water. If you are chronically dehydrated, you are literally starving yourself of your nutrients!

6. In the process of metabolism inside the cell, water breaks down and extracts the nutrients we need for energy. Chronic dehydration equals chronic fatigue.

7. Water is essential to rebuild every cell, tissue, and organ in our bodies. If we are chronically dehydrated, we are not regenerating properly.

Many of us experience thirst constantly. But when you get to the point where you don't experience thirst anymore, your dehydration is so severe your body has virtually stopped sending you the thirst signal. Dr. Batmanghelidj writes, "At this time, the 'dry mouth' is the only accepted sign of dehydration of the body. As I have explained, this signal is the last outward sign of extreme dehydration. The damage occurs at a level of persistent dehydration that does not necessarily demonstrate a 'dry mouth' signal . . . by the time you are thirsty, the damage to the body has already taken place." According to Dr. Batmanghelidj, by the time we feel thirst, the damage is done, so we must continually drink water. Let's face it. We are a water-dependent, water-burning machine, and this fuel must be replaced constantly.

With this in mind, I needed to find the best biological way—totally aligned with nature—to hydrate the body in a healthy way. I decided to look into the specific waters on the market. I went to back to Dr. Walker's books where he wrote that distilled water can remove the inorganic minerals out of the joints. I still had stiffness in my joints at that time, and I decided to drink nothing but distilled water to see how my body responded.

My joints definitely started to feel better, but after drinking the distilled water for a while, I started to feel twitching in my muscles and I was getting muscle cramps when I worked out at the gym. I also noticed that the vibrancy in my overall energy started to diminish. What was I missing? Distilled water was the cleanest and purest water in the world. However, because it was biologically dead, with the potential to usher toxins and minerals out of the body, I was experiencing mineral deficiencies. How would I replace those missing minerals and still drink pure water?

I studied Dr. Batmanghelidj's theories on the importance of salt in balancing the volume of water. He wrote, "The water we drink will keep the cell volume balanced and the salt we take will maintain the volume of water that is held outside the cells and in circulation."

Our bodily fluids are very close in biological makeup to seawater, and thus salt determines whether we can hold the hydration in the body. I'm not talking about unbalanced table salt, which dehydrates the body. As with many of my patients, every time I ate table salt, my joints hurt, my body swelled, and I felt tired. Table salt is imbalanced in its mineral content, and it dehydrates. I decided to look into different crude, unrefined salts, and when I started to use them, I noticed not only a huge jump in my energy, but they were actually helping my body hold hydration and helping to balance my bodily fluids. When I combined them with the use of different forms of ionic minerals, my body was adequately hydrated, and the signs of my mineral deficiencies mostly disappeared.

It's just not enough to drink the right kind of water. We have to look to the proper balance of our bodily fluids as well. Nobel Prize winner Dr. Alexis Carrell, gave us a great example of this when he was able to keep that chicken heart alive just by changing the fluids each day. He went on to state: "The cell is immortal. It is merely the fluid in which it floats that degenerates. Renew this fluid at regular intervals, give the cells what they require for nutrition, and as far as we know, the pulsation of life can go on forever."

Another great scientist and Nobel Prize winner, Dr. Albert Szent-Gyorgy, said, "Since the molecular structure of water is the essence of all life, the man who can control that structure in cellular systems will change the world."

Water Is Not Just Water

I wanted to hydrate my body with the best water I could find, but I was not happy with distilled water as an everyday medium. I noticed that I could drink certain bottled waters and I was still very thirsty; I wasn't getting hydrated enough. On the other hand, other bottled waters made me feel more hydrated, and I didn't have to drink as much. I wanted to know why certain waters were being absorbed by the cells and some were not. This obviously had to do with the water's structure.

I started to read about all kinds of waters, until my studies led me to what was called "structured/clustered" waters. I learned that how well the water is structured will determine how well it will be absorbed and enter the cells. There was a huge difference between the structure of bottled waters and the structured/clustered waters that were being produced by man. This led me to question how different the structure of the waters naturally occurring from the earth were as opposed to man-made waters that were called structured/clustered waters. Here is what I learned:

Tap water. This is referred to as "bound water" not only because it holds very little structure in its molecular makeup, but also because the tap water molecules become physically bound to other molecular structures. This makes it very difficult for this bound water to move freely through the walls of the cells.

Spring water. When some natural spring waters were tested, even though they contained significantly less pollutants than tap water, some of them were less hydrating than regular tap water!

Bottled water. Depending on the quality of the bottled water, it proved to be cleaner and safer to drink than tap water. In the bottled waters, the structuring and the mineral balance varied from water to water, which reflected in two ways. Some bottled waters hydrated better than others and since each had a different balance of minerals, each would feed the bodily fluids differently. I believed that drinking a variety and combination of waters was the smartest choice.

Distilled water. Distilled water was very hydrating. But because it is biologically dead (all the minerals have been removed), according to Dr. Walker, it can bind to other inorganic minerals and usher them out of the body. But as I observed my patients who were consuming only distilled water over a period of time, it seemed to usher out some beneficial minerals and elementals, which resulted in certain imbalances and muscle twitching.

Structured/clustered water. The original source of structured water was God-made. It came to humankind in the form of rainwater and snowflakes and was nature's most perfect hydrating gift. Unfortunately, over time, as the rainwater or snowflakes entered the increasingly toxic atmosphere, it lost its structure. This has had devastating effects on the human body.

There are two types of water in the body. Intercellular fluid is found outside the cell, and intracellular fluid is found inside the cell. Although both are vital for the proper functioning of the cell, the structure of our drinking water is vitally important to the amount of intracellular fluid that is maintained.

If our drinking water has too many large molecular structures, it will be unable to enter the doorway of the cell and will merely wash over and around the cell, leaving it dehydrated. If our drinking water is structured properly, though, it can enter the cell, creating a state of deep hydration. Structured or clustered water molecules are held together by small groups of rings. These molecules are shaped in just the right way so that their hexagonal structure can fit easily into and through the hexagonal channels in the cell membrane and enter the cell. This makes structured water very efficient in its hydrating effect.

If our cells are properly hydrated, they swell up, causing an anabolic healing reaction. This results in proper pH balance, increased fat burning capabilities, enhanced immunity against pathogens, and less free-radical damage. On the other hand, dehydrated cells encourage a catabolic state, which lends itself to increased inflammation, premature aging, and tissue degeneration.

Dehydration of the cells can force oxygen out of the cell, block the cell's ability to produce energy, damage the cell's DNA, increase cellular acidity, and cause cellular death. It is possible that too many accumulated cells that are severely dehydrated can lead to serious diseases.

Needless to say, the health of our cells, and therefore our bodies, depends on how much water can actually enter into our cells. As children, our bodies contain high amounts of clustered water, but unfortunately, as we get older, the level of unstructured water circulating in our bodies increases, diminishing metabolic functions and eliciting structural changes in our tissues.

I was looking for some specific factors, such as how well the water would hydrate the cells in the body and how diverse a range of ionic minerals and elementals that water would supply. My studies convinced me that I needed to test all the waters on my patients and myself to see which ones hydrated the body and blood most effectively. I used a dark-field microscope that could demonstrate changes in the blood.

As my patients and I drank these structured/clustered waters, the levels of our bodily hydration changed fairly rapidly. I noticed through other kinds of testing that the body's electrical conductivity also was improving. We tested tap water, which had poor hydration, and some popular bottled waters showed more improvement in hydration than tap water. But with most bottled waters, most people didn't feel completely hydrated, verified by their blood results. When we all drank structured/clustered waters, not only did our thirst disappear, but we had to drink less of this water to achieve hydration, which again was verified when we tested the blood. Why was that?

To keep it simple, water has an actual structure. The more structured/clustered the water, the lower the surface tension, which makes it electrically available to the cells of our body. The lower the surface tension, the wetter the water is and the more acceptable to our cells. My testing verified that the structure of the water determined how well our body was able to rehydrate. So far, structured/clustered water was winning the race by a long shot, but did one stand out above the others? That was not the case. There was no one water so complete that it would completely hydrate and constantly replace all the elements necessary to keep the bodily fluids in balance.

I started to use a combination of many structured/clustered waters as well as naturally occurring bottled waters. Also, I made sure to ingest different ionic mineral combos and varied unrefined salts at the same time. I started making my own waters, which I continue to do to this day. In fact, there is so much to learn about structured/clustered waters, ionic minerals, and unrefined salts, I put additional information on my Web site, continuing to educate the public. For my top choices for these waters, minerals, and salts, visit my Web site at www.Brantleycure.com

Masaru Emoto, author of the 2005 book *The Hidden Messages in Water*, writes, "Learning about water is like an exploration to discover how the cosmos works, and the crystals revealed through water are like the portal into another dimension. As we continued with our experiments in taking photographs of crystals, we found that we were setting out to climb the stars toward an understanding of the profound truths of the cosmos."

As you embark on rehydrating yourself in part two, "The Program for Balance," it would make sense to monitor your input versus output. In other words, if you're drinking and drinking and you are urinating very little, then you must increase your water intake very slowly. If you've been diagnosed with kidney problems or are taking diuretics or medications that affect your kidneys, be very cautious about increasing your water intake too quickly.

I urge you to take the next step. Your body has been crying out for the right kind of water for years, so give it a chance to heal. I believe that water is one of the most important keys to the health of the human body and that healing waters will become the medicine of the future. In chapter 13, "What to Drink and When," I will list a few personal water favorites. Bathe your body with the water of life and the benefits will be innumerable.

CHAPTER 10

My Study

I was convinced that most health problems were caused predominantly by incorrect eating, drinking, thinking, and living patterns, but I still needed answers as to what the body recognized as its correctly designed building blocks. Although I had strong opinions, I wanted to confirm what Creation considered correct and incorrect.

I theorized that if a food or a beverage was not acceptable, the body would provide an indicator that could be measured as an imbalance—causing other imbalances. I could then record specific foods and beverages possibly linked to the breakdowns in our health. Then we could learn to make the correct choices to achieve and maintain balance.

I decided to use myself and enlist some volunteer guinea pigs, but I used no one from my client base, since they were healthy by now and encouraged by how well they felt. Instead, I enlisted them to recruit their friends whom they considered healthy, who had seen their changes, and who were willing to volunteer.

Food Groups

In the end, I tested twelve people who ate from three different groups of foods. Everyone ate from the same food group at the same time. This was not a controlled study (it was too time-consuming and expensive to rent a facility and full-time testers), and my subjects were asked to just live their normal lives.

I began by giving each of my participants a list of foods they could or could not eat and drink for six to seven weeks. They could choose any food from their lists in the food group. At the end of the time period, they would be retested to report any changes. The tests were scheduled over a two-year period so I could establish a baseline reading on each individual. I did not separate or specify which foods were for breakfast, lunch, dinner, or snacks, leaving those decisions to the individual.

Food Group A (Standard American Diet)

The typical Standard American Diet (SAD). They could eat and drink all foods and beverages, even refined, processed, packaged, fast foods, and pasteurized dairy. The list included breads, cereals, toast, jelly, sugar, doughnuts, Danishes, muffins, Pop-Tarts, cakes, pies, ice cream, cookies, crackers, pasta, pancakes, and tortillas. They were allowed to eat from a can or a package, such as canned or processed vegetables, soups, fruit, meats, and any form of protein—cooked, fried, or baked—along with packaged and processed meats and deli meats, such as ham, bacon, pork, hamburger, steak, chicken, fish, and hot dogs.

Food Group B (Transitional Diet)

More limiting than Group A, this was an introduction into the arena of real foods directly from the earth and sea—fruits, vegetables, nuts, seeds, legumes, grains, potatoes, tubers, animal protein, and pasteurized dairy. Cooking was allowed, but no processed or refined foods or beverages. They drank bottled water, tea, coffee, and bottled pasteurized fruit and vegetable juices with no added sugar or sweeteners.

Food Group C (Predominantly Raw Diet)

Participants were required to eat at least 75 to 80 percent raw (no heating), directly from the land or the sea. The food was not to be altered, except the small amount (20 percent or less) that they could bake, steam, sear, or lightly cook in water. Included were fruits, nuts, vegetables, seeds, legumes, animal protein, raw dairy, and sprouted grains. No dried fruits. Only pure water and freshly squeezed fruit and vegetable juices were allowed.

Just before the testing, as I interviewed people who considered them-selves healthy, I learned that they had different physical complaints, excluding chronic injuries. They collectively admitted that they felt like falling asleep after most meals and wanted more energy, unaware that the energy roller coaster during the day, sleeping badly and awakening tired, was not normal. I found it interesting that because everyone had been living this way consistently, they never expected their bodies to respond differently.

Testing and Evaluation Methods

I used the following six testing and evaluation methods:

- Food and blood sugar testing
- Electrodermal screening (EAV)
- Live blood analysis (dark-field microscope)
- Applied kinesiology
- PH testing
- Client interviews, response, and feedback

Testing results with each group follow each method.

Food Blood Sugar Testings

Participants would take a baseline reading of their blood sugar levels before meals and measure them again every fifteen to twenty minutes for the first two hours for changes in blood sugar levels.

Test Results
Food Group A (Standard American Diet). Blood sugar (blood glucose) levels rose high and rapidly. Consuming these refined and processed foods, laced with an overabundance of refined sugar, set off a myriad of imbalances. Recognizing a dangerous condition, the body was forced to engage its emergency rescue systems to force sugars down.

Food Group B (Transitional Diet). Blood sugar rose slower and test subjects did not feel a quick rush of energy at the start of a meal or a sudden drop after the meal. Overall, blood glucose levels did not swing as fast. The subjects were more stable but remained imbalanced.

Food Group C (Predominantly Raw Diet). Blood sugar rose slowly. It rose too quickly or too high only if the participant drank too much freshly squeezed fruit juice too rapidly. Everyone reported no postmeal slump and sleepiness, no quick rushes of energy at the start and a sudden drop of energy after the meal. No one reported the terrible roller-coaster effect with their blood sugars.

Electrodermal Screening (EAV)

This system, developed by Reinhold Voll, M.D., in the 1940s, can detect dysfunctions and infection in the individual acupuncture meridian systems of the body. When an electrical current running through an electrode is placed on that specific meridian, it can record a specific electrical resistance at that acupuncture point or specific meridian. A disturbance or infection causing a deviation from the normal reading, either too high or too low, could give me information that the organ or system within that meridian was in an unbalanced and unhealthy state. The practitioner, using probes applied to specific acupuncture meridian points on the skin of the hands and feet, gathered information by reading the electrical feedback, such as energy losses in that system, possible toxicity, inflammations, irritations, and possible degeneration.

Test Results
Food Group A (Standard American Diet). In the first test immediately after the meal, subjects registered high readings at most meridian points, indicating overworking or overstimulation in each body system. By the second test, subjects were vacillating slightly but mostly switching to low readings, indicating an extreme loss of energy in that system. The imbalances created various strained and overworked systems in the body, eventually wearing them down. The third test found almost every system registering fatigue and a loss of energy.

Food Group B (Transitional Diet). In the first test immediately after the meal, subjects vacillated between high and low readings at most meridian points, indicating overworking or overstimulation in each body system, but nowhere near the extremes in Food Group A. By the second test, subjects vacillated between some high readings and switching to lower readings, indicating loss of energy in that system. Again, the low readings were nowhere near the extremes in those eating Group A foods. Mild fluctuations between highs and lows indicated that these foods were not stressing the body nearly as much, with some imbalances improving and their overall energy becoming far more stable. By the third test, almost every system in most subjects registered a slight loss of energy or fatigue.

Food Group C (Predominantly Raw Diet). In the first test immediately after the meal, subjects had little vacillation between higher and lower readings in most meridian points, indicating far less overworking or overstimulation. The second and third tests indicated little fluctuations or imbalances.

Live Blood Analysis (Dark-Field Microscope)

The blood microscopist would take a drop of blood from the subject's finger and examine it under a dark-field microscope that gives different images with a change of lenses. It reflects many different factors in the blood and the plasma. Information about the health of the red and white blood cells can be gathered, as well as readings of blood and plasma, whether the cells have been damaged by free radicals, and whether their dehydrated and toxic environments are damaging them. It can also show some nutritional deficiencies, microbes, parasites, and fungi. In addition, it allows observation of blood movement, which can indicate the activity, health, and vibrancy of the cells. These are just some of the many things that this test can observe about the current condition of only the blood.

Test Results

Food Group A (Standard American Diet). The longer the subjects stayed on this bad diet, the more their blood profiles degenerated, with increased yeast proliferation (*Candida albicans fungus*). Stagnation increased, blood slowly lost vitality, and we detected hormonal stress, parasites, microbes, and vitamin deficiencies. The oxygen-deprived blood cells became sluggish and stuck together, indicating a loss of electrical life. This group was dehydrated, and the yeast overproliferation from excess sugar in the blood caused fatigue, bloating, gas, intestinal discomfort, and bowel problems. I detected uric acid crystals caused by dehydration. I also detected blood cells sticking together (a condition called rouleau), an extremely unhealthy state. Nutritional deficiencies also were detected.

Food Group B (Transitional Diet). Subjects exhibited a slow but fairly large decrease in yeast proliferation (*Candida albicans fungus*) compared to those in group A. The movement of red blood cells improved noticeably; they became far more vibrant and active. They still needed lots of improvement, but there were fewer opportunistic microbes than for those eating Group A foods, indicating too much undigested material and toxic waste. Hormonal stress improved a little, more in women than men; vitamin deficiencies were still detected; and the blood cells, although less sluggish, still stuck together. Dehydration improved but remained a significant problem. Leukocytosis also was detected in those in Group B, since the body actually looks at cooked food as a foreign invader.

Food Group C (Predominantly Raw Diet). The longer they ate pure raw foods, the more their blood profiles improved. Everyone exhibited a large decrease in yeast proliferation (*Candida albicans fungus*), which I attribute to eliminating most grains, potatoes, and most legumes unless sprouted or slightly cooked. Although some stagnation or lack of activity of the red blood cells remained, it improved slightly in the overall group. The blood became more vibrant and active compared with the blood in those eating any amount of cooked foods. There were fewer opportunistic microbes in the blood tested from eating Group C foods than in the blood of those eating Group A foods, indicating far less processed undigested material and toxic waste in the blood.

Applied Kinesiology

In his 2002 book *Alternative Medicine: The Definitive Guide*, Burton Goldberg says, "Applied Kinesiology employs a simple strength resistance test on a specific indicator muscle, related to the organ or part of the body being tested. If the muscle tests strong (maintaining its resistance), it indicates health. A weak test means infection or dysfunction."

Robert Blaich, D.C., of Denver, Colorado, a leading expert in applied kinesiology, says, "Because of the close clinical relationship between specific muscle dysfunction and related organ or gland dysfunction, applied Kinesiology can identify and treat a wide variety of health problems, whether they originate in a muscle, gland, or organ."

Test Results

Food Group A (Standard American Diet). All general body points continually fluctuated and progressively weakened depending on the severity of the amount of refined sugar and processed flour products and drinks consumed. This diet created imbalances in most meridian systems.

Food Group B (Transitional Diet). Most of the general body points, such as the pancreas, kidneys, and adrenals, improved in all test subjects. I attribute this to withdrawing from refined sugar, flour products, and heavily processed meats. Foods eaten in this form were not creating as many imbalances as foods in the highly refined diet of Food Group A (Standard American Diet).

Food Group C (Predominantly Raw Diet). Eating foods directly from the earth in their untouched and raw form gave the strongest overall body testing. The pancreas, kidneys, and adrenals slowly improved in all test subjects, since raw foods were not creating nearly as many imbalances as a highly refined diet or a diet of predominantly cooked foods.

PH Testing

PH testing, which I have previously covered, is a way to look at the body's biochemistry and determine the acid/alkaline state of balance of certain body fluids. When the pH is out of balance, enzyme systems work poorly, nutrients are not absorbed as well, and you can become undernourished, fatigued, and vulnerable to outside invaders. Certain types of pH testing also can measure imbalanced sugar, salt, and protein levels, as well as other things.

Test Results

Food Group A (Standard American Diet). These foods created wild imbalances in the pH testing, the most telling indicator being the constant tendency to throw everyone's body into acidosis and symptoms of extreme mineral deficiencies.

Food Group B (Transitional Diet). These foods created imbalances in the pH but did not swing as wildly as for those eating Group A foods. There was a slower tendency to turn acidic, although everyone remained somewhat acidic.

Food Group C (Predominantly Raw Diet). Eating group C raw foods had the best overall balancing effect on the pH. Although there were still imbalances in everyone's pH, these foods did not cause the wild radical swings that resulted from eating Group A foods. Those in Group C also improved when compared with those eating Group B foods.

Client Interviews, Response, and Feedback

I recorded my clients' responses to eating food from these specific groups—if they liked eating them, how they felt before and after a meal, and how they felt each week thereafter. How did these foods affect their moods? Did their overall energy change? How was their energy throughout the day?

Food Group A (Standard American Diet). The subjects all had radical energy fluctuations, staying in a cycle of having to manipulate to produce quick energy after a radical drop. The subjects all remarked that they never realized how addicted they were to sugar and other stimulants, like caffeine, simply to function. The roller-coaster effect on their energy swung them into high and low moods, and many of them got sick consistently.

Food Group B (Transitional Diet). They had fewer quick highs and quick lows, and overall their energy was more stable and they were less fatigued and not depressed as often. They did not get sick as often, either, which surprised everyone.

Food Group C (Predominantly Raw Diet). The overall opinion was that everyone admitted they felt far better when eating Group C foods than they did when eating Group A or Group B foods. In fact, subjects said the overall effect of eating Group C foods vs. eating Group A foods was drastically different. They said they were consistently happier than before, and they did not get sick as often as when they ate foods from Group A or Group B.

In my clinical practice, I already discovered that if certain factors were used regularly, my clients could return to a state of balance. If they continued applying these factors regularly, they could remain balanced and in optimal health. As noted, disease cannot live in a balanced and healthy body.

Eating predominantly raw food had already proved successful with my clients—I did this study to record the human body's actual responses. I observed, however, that the people in my studies were still missing certain things that kept them from achieving balance and completely regaining their health.

In reviewing their reactions, I then realized that I should conduct a small study using all the pieces that I had discovered all at one time. This small group ate foods only from Group C, and they made sure they were adequately hydrated at all times with structured/clustered waters and ion-rich waters. They supported both their current and inherited weaknesses with Group C foods and my herbal formulas, making sure they consumed a smorgasbord of nutrients on a meal-to-meal basis. They also detoxified and desolidified the years of toxins with my herbal formulas. Over a fairly short time, everyone in this small group found that their symptoms disappeared and they were able to regain their health. The beauty of eating and drinking from Mother Nature's table!

The Missing Factors

1. Even though Group C was heading in the right direction, eating directly from the ground and keeping it in the correct form, their unfortunate patterns of eating the same narrow choice of foods repetitively was not giving them access to the broad range of nutrients their bodies needed regularly. In essence, they were still nutritionally starving.

2. Eating processed and refined foods (Group A) caused excesses of the wrong things, such as toxic wastes, to enter the body. These created imbalances and constantly stressed all systems. It also forced the body to compensate for these excesses by stealing from its own reserves to restore balance.

3. If those inherited weaknesses were not supported and corrected, those weaknesses could contribute to their imbalances.

4. If someone in their family smoked, those in the study needed to work on supporting their own lungs and removing heavy metals from their body.

5. If either parent had a blood sugar weakness, those in the study needed to support their own pancreas, liver, adrenals, and kidneys.

6. One other factor was missing: desolidification. I will discuss this soon.

Imbalances Corrected

When Group C clients' specific imbalances were corrected, the overall body finally returned to a state of balance, and health problems or diseases disappeared. Here were some stunning results:

1. Rehydration of every organ, gland, and tissue balanced their cells and maximized their operating output.

2. The blood became more vibrant, less toxic, more oxygenated, healthier, and more balanced.

3. The pH of the body fluid returned to balance, which kept the cells highly oxygenated. Cancer, viruses, unhealthy fungus, bad microbes, and parasites cannot live in this kind of environment.

4. The organs, glands, and tissue, once cleared of the clogging toxic material, returned to a state of health and balance.

5. The meridian systems of the body regained their balance and worked in harmony.

PART TWO

The Program for Balance

CHAPTER 11

The Brantley Road Map to Balance

I now understood what people needed to do to raise their energy, diminish their cravings, and restore and maintain balance. But I knew I could not work with everyone at the same time. So I had to devise a system that would give all the steps necessary to regain and maintain balance. I call this the Brantley road map to balance. Whether you eat junk food or you eat raw, whether you are sick or healthy, this road map will improve your overall health and well-being.

Guidelines

1. *Hydration.* Slowly rehydrate the body and maintain balance at all times. Also, constantly feed the body fluids.
2. *Slowly eliminate processed foods.* You will be shown in the upcoming chapters how to make a slow and safe transition from processed foods.

3. *Supply what you need and eat broadly at all times.* Your job is to supply your body as broad a range as possible of the correct nutrients in the correct form as often as possible. Even with my clients who ate foods from Group C, I still had to help them regain balance and maintain it. I helped them supply all of the correct biological elements in the correct form, from a variety of concentrated food sources. What a great insurance policy! Then their body can pick and choose anything it needs for repair, balance, and restoration, providing the necessary building blocks to restore, regenerate, and rebuild. When someone gives the body the same narrow range of nutritionally deficient foods all the time, it eventually catches up with them.

4. *Break conditioned patterns; support and rebuild the weakened areas.* I constantly helped people break generational patterns that had created a weakness or could influence that weakness to continue. For example, if diabetes or blood sugar problems, heart problems, or cancer were prevalent in a person's family lineage, the person might already have this problem or at least be vulnerable to it due to family eating and drinking patterns. When that was the case, we would automatically work on that weakness, breaking the learned dietary pattern that created it while supporting the particular weakened area. I then made specific herbal formulas to support those weakened areas that ran in their family.

5. *Detoxify and desolidify.* Did you ever wonder why you can't digest the same type of foods that you used to? And why is it that now, when you eat a small amount of that same type of food, you gain weight? It's because your body and your organs are not working up to the same capacity anymore. They are tired, overworked, and clogged. Slowly soften and remove the years of toxins, poisons, inorganics, trans-fatty acids, heavy metals, and hardened mucus with undigested foods that block and clog each system. Solidification creates blockages that do not allow the nutrients to be properly metabolized and absorbed into the cells. Years of trapped material can eventually clog and greatly inhibit the intestinal tract, the liver and gallbladder, the kidneys, adrenals, pancreas, and brain, even affecting the tissue level of the body. These things are constantly causing irritation, which eventually leads to inflammation. And inflammation is the body's first step toward ill health and disease. Blockages can be created to such an extent that these systems eventually have a hard time doing their jobs.

Start slowly, detoxifying one system at a time. Each system must be cleansed repeatedly, at specific intervals, to clear up the many years of waste trapped and causing the blockages. These detoxification and desolidification programs will be explained in chapter 15.

6. *Take herbal formulas to:*
   - Detoxify
   - Desolidify
   - Maintain
   - Support and rebuild weakened areas
   - Supply a wide range of nutrients

Remember, I did not cure my clients. They cured themselves and returned to a state of balance by the choices they made. You can cure yourself, too. Living in a state of balance is your choice.

Once you begin, don't worry if you fall off the program. Just start back right where you are and remember that everyone is in a different place, so don't compare yourself with anyone else. Once you apply these principles for a while, they will become second nature.

Let's review all the vital keys that you need to follow if you want to achieve balance and therefore optimal health.

Brantley's Twelve Keys to Balance

1. Properly hydrate yourself throughout the day with the right kinds of structured/clustered water and/or mineral-rich bottled water.

2. Break the incorrect generational and societal eating patterns by following proper eating programs.

3. Identify and support your current problems.

4. Support and rebuild your inherited propensity for weakened areas in your family heritage.

5. Every morning and before meals, drink lemon and water.

6. First stop putting into your body what shouldn't be there. Then eat a smorgasbord of nutrients in their correct form, on a meal-to-meal basis, every day of your life. Let your body pick and choose what it needs.

7. Eliminate table salt and use only balanced, unrefined sea salt.

8. Eat mostly raw foods, untouched, the way they were created by nature.

9. Chew your food until it is liquid before swallowing.

10. Take enzymes before and with cooked food.

11. Try not to drink with meals, but if you do, have a small amount of room-temperature water only. Hot and cold drinks inhibit digestion.

12. Detoxify, decalcify, and desolidify.

If you are diligent and committed to changing your patterns and turning your health around, follow my keys every day for the rest of your life. There are no quick fixes and no magic bullets. Your body is just waiting for the chance to heal. Do the work, give it some time, and soon you will not believe how well you feel. My twelve keys will lead you to vibrant health. So many of my clients throughout the years have followed my principles and have been triumphant in their battle against serious diseases. Once you follow all my guidelines including detoxification, decalcification, and desolidification, it will help reverse inflammation and prevent it from occurring anywhere in your body.

CHAPTER 12

A Little Inspiration

Now that I've laid out an entire program to transform your eating patterns, I hope you'll follow my guidelines for the rest of your life! After all, this is an insurance policy for you and your family—a program all about *prevention*. The point is to do the work so you don't get diagnosed with a serious disease. Please don't wait until it's too late to reverse it.

One of my clients was fortunate. He changed his eating patterns out of desperation—his life was on the line and he quickly discovered he had no choice. In truth, none of us does. I believe if you don't change the way you eat and drink today, you're risking your life and the lives of your children.

In my clinical practice, all too often I've seen the haunting look of regret on clients' faces when they realized they could have saved their own lives if they'd known enough to throw out all their nonfoods. Although it's a good start, it isn't enough just to read this book. You need to take action and always remember:

You are the cause and you are the cure.

Please use Howie's story for additional inspiration to change what you put in your mouth forever! Howie did just that, and he was fortunate he got to me in time. Now it's your time to follow my programs to ensure great health for you and those you love.

Howie Klein's Story

Howie Klein, president of Reprise Records, was stunned when he was diagnosed with prostate cancer, since he'd been following a supposedly healthy diet for years. A vegetarian since his teenage years, a man who had explored macrobiotics, Howie was a former all-natural chef in Amsterdam. He did admit that he ate too much sugar. When he moved back to the States, although he avoided fast food, he let his healthy diet slip as he reintroduced cooked fish and chicken into his diet. Finally, as president of a large record company, Howie was crushed under twenty-four-hour stress, and he ate without particularly reflecting on what he was eating.

One look in the irises of Howie's eyes told me he'd done a lot of drugs in his day. The truth was that he'd stopped in 1969, but after so much prior destructive behavior, a diagnosis of prostate cancer was not so strange or mysterious.

Howie was willing to follow my protocols meticulously, with no fooling around. He already drank no coffee, he'd quit soft drinks in the late 1960s, he'd never smoked cigarettes, and he had hardly ever drunk beer. That was all a plus, making it easy for me to tell him no sugar or flour. Eager to lose weight as well as heal his cancer, he immediately gave up pizza, flour, sugar, and everything else that was doing him no earthly good.

In six months, Howie lost forty pounds. "Wow," his friends commented, "you lost half of you!" He was thrilled, realizing that the doctors had dealt with only a part of him while I addressed his entire body and mind. In fact, losing weight was tangential in dealing with his health problems, but still a part of the whole. As a result of cleansing, the bottoms of his feet stopped itching (he hadn't told me about them until they got better), and his thirteen-year case of dandruff disappeared.

Most important was how much better he felt. Howie began to exercise more; he got twenty minutes of sunshine on his face each day, and he walked everywhere. He increased his water intake, took my anti-cancer formulas, ate and drank as I instructed, and restored his body back to balance. Since disease cannot live in a healthy body, his cancer was suddenly homeless, and Howie felt like a million bucks. He stopped catching colds and avoided catching the flu, while most people with whom he worked got really sick.

Howie's internist was open to his healing, fascinated with my protocols and suggestions. His urologist, on the other hand, was an angry man who, in Howie's words, "was enraged that I'd gone outside the medical protocols." He considered surgery as the only cure, no matter how clean Howie's tests came out. Testing revealed that Howie's cancer was gone.

"I think of my doctor when I wake up at six every morning and I jump out of bed feeling great, ready to take on the world," Howie told me. He made my natural-food philosophy his own, and he takes my products daily for maintenance and cancer prevention and as an elixir for his overall health. I was gratified when he told me a true story about having Howard Dean, a doctor and former governor of Vermont, to his home for breakfast in 2003.

"As a donor to the Democratic Party," Howie said, "I was interested in Howard Dean's presidential run, since he seemed like a progressive kind of guy. I served him what I eat—half a papaya stuffed with blueberries, ground-up flax seeds, and some fresh juice mixed with greens. Apparently Governor Dean still tells his friends how wonderful it was to eat light and not start his day with a bellyful of bacon, eggs, white toast, jam, and a barrel of caffeine."

They discussed the possibility of addressing the disastrous American health system. Dean was enthusiastic, and when he left, Howie had made a new friend with whom he'd shared his newfound vitality and the miracle of Creation.

Now it's time for you and your family to get to work. What are your challenges? Are you constantly in pain? Do you have a chronic illness that has plagued you for years? Are you exhausted, depressed, and overweight? Can you really afford to wait any longer? None of us is getting any younger. The clock is ticking. Why live the rest of your life suffering from symptoms that your body could heal if given half a chance? The following chapters could save or change your life. If you apply all the principles in my programs for balance, you will feel much better in twelve weeks than you ever have in your entire life.

CHAPTER 13

What to Drink and When

If you're serious about regaining your health, it is imperative to drink pure, balanced and structured/clustered water. The following two-week program of rehydration revolves around drinking this kind of water. This will be an adjustment period in which you are setting yourself up for what you will do every day for the rest of your life! Let's keep it simple.

How Much Water Should I Drink Daily?

You should be drinking at least 50 to 75 percent of your body weight in ounces per day. That means if you weigh 150 pounds, you need to drink 75 to 112 ounces of pure water per day. Here are some rules to start your rehydration process:

1. If you rarely drink water, you need to slowly work up to your daily intake. Start with the amount you're already drinking and add one more eight-ounce glass per day. This may take you a little longer to fully hydrate your system, but it is detrimental to drown your cells with too much water, too fast, as it creates imbalances.

2. Approximately twenty to thirty minutes before your meal, drink a full glass of water to prepare the body and the stomach for digestion. This is a great time to add your enzymes. This water also will rehydrate the mucus layer of the stomach and help keep the stomach acid from irritating or possibly burning the stomach tissue. It will also help protect against acid reflux. Hydrating the pancreas and liver, the organs involved in digestion, ensures that these organs will work more efficiently. Try squeezing the juice of a quarter of a fresh organic lemon into the water to help stimulate digestion.

3. Do not drink with meals if possible. This dilutes the power and effectiveness of not only your internal enzymes that you have secreted but also the enzyme capsules you have taken. All hot and cold beverages inactivate enzymes and block proper digestion. Chewing until your food is liquid will help any thirst cravings while you eat. Remember, teeth are for chewing, and your stomach doesn't have teeth. If you absolutely can't go without drinking during a meal, during this two-week transition period, you can have four ounces of room-temperature water while eating. Try not to drink for at least an hour after your meal.

4. Make sure you drink water every half hour. Don't wait two hours and drink it all at once. You should be drinking twice every hour, so you need to figure out your weight and the amount of ounces of water you need to drink on an hour-to-hour basis. Never forget that you are a water-burning machine. If you exercise heavily, compensate for the water loss by drinking water every fifteen to twenty minutes during exercise periods.

5. Make sure that you are using clean, purified water to rehydrate your system. I shudder to think that anyone would pour themselves a glass of water from the tap. Please do not do this! Here are some facts:

   In 1993, over 400,000 people in Milwaukee became sick from contaminated tap water and at least 104 died. The shocking fact was that at this same time, the Milwaukee water system met all state and federal health standards.

   In 1992, the Environmental Protection Agency (EPA) tested 8,100 municipal water systems and found 10 percent of them with unsafe levels of lead. These 819 water systems distributed water to over 30 million people.

The horror stories go on and on. What is in your tap water right now? On a day-to-day basis, none of us really knows. So now what?

I would suggest that you use a clean and reputable bottled water. In Los Angeles, my patients in the clinic prepare their bottled water by adding a pinch of sea salt and a squeeze of organic lemon juice for better hydration. They shake their bottle vigorously for a few seconds before drinking. Some suggestions are Fiji Water, Hawaiian Water, or Iceland Water, but you should do your own homework on the bottled water that you decide to drink on a regular basis. I find these brands to be more naturally structured and therefore more hydrating.

In my opinion and based on exhaustive research over the years, the very best and safest structured/clustered waters are not available on the retail shelf. If you are interested in those waters, please visit my Web site at www.Brantleycure.com.

Lemon Aid

Lemon is one of the most powerful foods for supporting the digestive organs, since it helps to turn on the body's energy and to cleanse and activate the liver. Upon rising, drink 8 ounces of the preparation mentioned above (bottled or structured water with a pinch of sea salt and a squeeze of organic lemon juice).

Lemon is one of the only foods with the same kind of energy as the liver. The liver and the lemon contain what is called anionic (negatively charged ionic) energy, while most foods contain a cationic (positive charged ionic) energy. In this way, the anionic lemon helps to feed, support, and turn on the anionic liver while refueling it. In chemistry, it is the coming together of these two opposing forces that creates energy.

When the cationic foods arrive in the body, the opposing forces bump into one another, causing a beneficial energy explosion—one of the ways we derive energy from food. When you drink lemon juice and water first thing in the morning, you successfully turn on your liver, warming up the engine, preparing the liver to support the digestive process. The juice of a lemon also stimulates the liver to kick on the digestive juices. If you ate dinner too late the night before, lemon juice first thing in the morning helps stimulate the digestive juices to enter the blood and clean up the debris, the undigested food particles.

To exponentially increase the cleansing action, add to the lemon and water a pinch of cayenne pepper, a small amount of freshly grated ginger, and/or an optional half teaspoon of grade B organic maple syrup. During your detoxification period, this is a very effective cleansing drink to start off your day, as it is great for your circulation. Even if you stick with simple lemon juice in water, the lemon juice itself has a very powerful cleansing effect. Lemons are full to the brim with vitamin C and bioflavonoids, which are plant derivatives with antioxidant and anti-inflammatory properties.

When I was a teenager studying the pH theories of Carey Reams, I read that he loved the lemon's powerful effect on the body's biochemistry and pH levels. The lemon is high in potassium, one of the top five macrominerals essential for health and well-being. I suggest you drink lemon and water twenty to thirty minutes before each meal.

Signs to Watch for as You Rehydrate Your System

1. Sometimes when you start to rehydrate, your body can swell in certain places. This should disappear as you slowly rehydrate yourself. Just be consistent and be patient and have faith that it is working.

2. As an added insurance policy, make sure you remineralize yourself at the same time you drink water. Finding a broad-based and balanced liquid mineral combination is tricky, because you can't use any old kind of cheap liquid minerals from a health food store. I spent years of my life tracking down the best sources, so why reinvent the wheel? There is no reason to make it harder for your body to function by feeding it minerals that are not up to speed, which is why I included a list of my favorite ionic minerals on my Web site (www.Brantleycure.com).

3. Watch the color of your urine. It should be almost colorless or light yellow. If you take a synthetic vitamin supplement or a separate vitamin B complex, your urine will tend to be bright yellow. It would be best to stop taking your multivitamins and your B complex for the next couple of weeks so you can accurately judge your urine color. I don't believe synthetic vitamins should be used at all.

4. If you notice that your urine is darker than usual, you can be sure your body is not being adequately hydrated. You may have done a good job of drinking your water one day and then forgot to drink every hour the next day because you were too busy. The body doesn't care how busy you are or what kind of work deadline you are under. All it knows is that it needs to be replenished with water constantly throughout the day or it can't do its job properly. If it can't do its job, you will suffer the consequences!

5. If you have trouble sleeping, drink a glass of water. Then put a pinch of balanced unrefined salt on the tip of your tongue and let it dissolve. Do not touch your tongue to the top of your palate, because the salt can irritate. This also can work for migraine headaches, but substitute a glass of cold water instead—the *only* time I suggest using cold water.

6. If you have a weight problem, your food cravings may be a sign of thirst, not hunger! Your body may be mixing up signals. Over the years, many of my clients reported that with adequate hydration, their food cravings diminished.

7. If you have an extremely toxic body, it will most likely be quite challenging to rehydrate, but don't get discouraged. You are only just beginning, and your body will be ecstatic when an adequate amount of water dilutes and washes away years of accumulated toxins and debris.

By slowly hydrating your body, the perfect first step, you are embarking on the process of detoxification. You have to start somewhere, and without rehydration, it will be impossible to achieve optimal health. The results of consistent hydration, although a seemingly simple step, are not to be believed.

Dr. Batmanghelidj treated thousands of his patients with water alone, as countless "diseases" unable to be reversed with pharmaceuticals eventually disappeared. I have also seen many miracles with water, so take these next two weeks and dedicate yourself to this process. As demonstrated by so many of my clients' stories, compliance can either make you or break you. In the end, you are the only one with the power to turn your health around.

Action Steps

1. Start the morning with eight ounces of pure water and the juice of a quarter of an organic lemon.

2. Drink 50 to 75 percent of your body weight in ounces every day.

3. Always drink room-temperature water.

4. Don't drink with your meals. Wait at least one hour after a meal to resume drinking pure water.

5. Twenty to thirty minutes before meals, drink a glass of water with lemon. If lemons are not available, drink water anyway. This is a good time to take plant enzymes.

6. Drink water every thirty minutes, and never go more than one hour without pure water.

7. Follow this protocol every day. Compliance is everything!

Besides oxygen, water is the most important element in your body's overall health and well-being. You can live quite a while without food, but you can live only a short period of time without water. In her book *Nutrition in Perspective*, Patricia Kreutler writes, "A person will die within 3–4 days without water."

Remember that you're establishing this new drinking pattern for your lifetime, since you can't ever afford to go even half a day without hydrating yourself! You can no longer use the excuse that you forgot to drink, or that you don't like the taste of water, or that you were just too busy. You *cannot* substitute any other beverage for pure water, even if you think that beverage is natural. When I drink fresh juices, I always keep up with my pure-water intake. Just because you drink fresh juices doesn't mean you can stop drinking water.

To avoid confusion, I want to make sure to direct you to the best bottled and structured/clustered waters. I still spend countless hours doing research on the ever-changing water market, and I want you to benefit from my findings. Please visit my Web site, www.Brantleycure.com, where I will help you choose the waters that are right for your body.

CHAPTER 14

What to Eat and When

Congratulations on taking the first step toward your renewed health by rehydrating your system. Now it's time for the next two weeks of your program. Many people invariably get up too late, take a shower, throw on their clothes, dump some processed cereal, sugar, and pasteurized milk in a bowl, smear margarine and jelly on toast, slam it all down, and run out the door, coffee in hand—the fastest, easiest breakfast possible. Or maybe you stop at your local Starbucks for a sweet Mocha Grande and a sugary scone. You've trashed yourself before you even arrive at work, as your adrenals pound under a caffeine surge and your blood sugar climbs through the roof. You've thrown off your biochemistry and started to turn your body acidic, forcing oxygen out of the cells, setting the stage for viruses, cancer, and bacteria to proliferate. You have to dip into your reserve energy, since the coffee has further dehydrated your already dehydrated cells. If you've become a card-carrying member of the Pop-Tart, toast, and bagel club, you've slowly but surely been tearing down your body every morning, setting yourself up for a major downfall. You've consumed a load of dead, processed, devitalized, nutritionally deficient, health-destroying so-called foods, starting your day by traveling down the road to imbalance.

Remember, health is all about balance—eating balanced and nourishing daily meals that contain the broadest range of vitamins, macro- and microminerals, amino acids, essential fatty acids, saturated fat, protein, and enzymes in the correct form.

Let's use the upcoming weeks to totally transform your breakfast experience. For now, don't worry about lunch or dinner. First develop great breakfast habits before you proceed to the next meal. Start by reading Guidelines for Eating a Balanced Meal.

Guidelines for Eating a Balanced Meal

Note the following:

- Be conscious of everything you put in your mouth.

- Twenty to thirty minutes before your meal, drink pure water and lemon to prepare your stomach for digestion.

- Eat raw fruits and vegetables to rebalance your pH levels.

    Eating cooked foods for a lifetime has so depleted our body's enzyme reserves, we can't get away with eating the same foods we did when we were kids. I suggest you eat lots of raw foods, because their enzymes are intact. If you do eat partially cooked foods, you must take living plant enzymes before, during, and after that meal. I always take plant enzymes if I eat partially cooked foods. This protects my enzyme reserves, protects my immune system, and helps fight the aging process. Don't forget that cooking food destroys enzymes and vitamins while it damages essential fatty acids and saturated fats, rendering them dangerous to the body.

    On the other hand, when you eat raw and live foods that are unprocessed, coming directly from the earth, you'll derive more energy from your food than it takes to digest it.

- Eat like the wild animals—directly from the earth. They don't change the form of food they eat, and they have great health. This means you should *not eat any* processed or junk food that will load your body with toxins.

- Choose foods that don't create a quick rise and fall in your blood sugar. Avoid *all* refined grain products—bread, pasta, tortilla chips, and pastries.

- Proper food combinations ensure an easy digestive process. Don't eat protein, grains, and starches together, since the enzymes used to digest each of these foods employ opposite digestive pH mediums to break them down, slowing digestion and creating fermentation. That means no meat and potatoes and no sandwiches—because you can't eat protein and bread at the same time. Fruits should be eaten thirty minutes before a meal or one to two hours after. Eat whole sprouted grains with vegetables.

- We all tend to eat the same foods over and over, but if you don't branch out, you can't get your needed nutrition. An iceberg lettuce salad with tomatoes and cucumbers will not give you everything you need from the vegetable kingdom. Make sure your diverse food choices contain the broadest range of easily assimilated vitamins, minerals, amino acids, essential fatty acids, saturated fat, protein, and enzymes in their live, unaltered form.

- Chew your food until it is liquid, so the food sources can deliver the energy and nutrition upon which we depend daily. If you must drink with a meal, make it a small amount of the highest-quality and balanced room-temperature water.

- Stay away from all hydrogenated oils. Unless the oil is raw, don't buy it or cook with it. Lightly blanch food in a small amount of water and herbs. Then add your raw oils after blanching. If you must, lightly sear your food in raw coconut oil or cold-pressed extra-virgin olive oil.

- Use no refined table salt. Only high-quality, balanced, and unrefined sea salts or unrefined and balanced mineral and herb salts are acceptable.

- Buy organic vegetables and fruits as well as hormone-free meats if your budget and location permit. If not, buy a natural spray in your local supermarket that can wash off herbicides and pesticides.

- Do not eat desserts after a meal, especially sugary ones after protein.

- Throw out your microwave oven. I know this is a sad day for many of you, but here are the real facts about food cooked in the microwave. When you take the food out of the microwave, I believe it keeps on cooking! When that nuked food hits your stomach at such a high temperature, it destroys not only the nutritional content of your food, but also, in my opinion, it could possibly cause tissue damage. The only thing your microwave is good for is to anchor your boat.

A Vitamin Is Not Just a Vitamin

Many of us take vitamins and minerals at breakfast, but you may not understand the difference between supplements from your local drugstore and what you buy at the health food store. There are three kinds of vitamin supplements on the market today. Some are food-based, but many vitamin and mineral supplements are extracted from a food or made in a lab, unable to give anywhere near the benefits of eating natural foods. Isolating and extracting vitamins from a food source throws the body into a quandary, since vitamins and minerals are team players, not solo acts.

Your body will view synthetic vitamin supplements as foreign invaders, with no idea what to do with them. The synthetic supplement will use too much of your energy and enzymes to digest it, becoming yet another manipulated substance of which the body needs to rid itself. Others, however, are made in a lab. Manufacturers sometimes use petrochemicals to extract a particular vitamin from a food source. Nice, huh? The supplement you thought would benefit you is putting more strain on your already tired and worn-out system. Test this theory by putting your vitamin supplement in the oven at 425 degrees for thirty minutes. If your house smells like chemicals or the pill turns a scary shade of black or brown, the extracting agent is not something to feed your body.

A vitamin supplement from the drugstore is another scary story, since the lab vitamin people argue that a vitamin is a vitamin. Why pay more at a health food store, they brainwash us, when you can buy a thousand vitamin tablets right here for practically nothing? They're right. You can get them for practically nothing because you're getting less than nothing in the long run. In fact, it's doing you more harm than good, since most cheap drugstore lab vitamins contain dead chemicals. If you cook a peach pit for a day and then you plant it in the ground, I guarantee you'll starve to death before you see a tree grow from that dead peach pit.

In my opinion, dead synthetic vitamin supplements should be tossed in the garbage along with all your health-destroying medications. I am *not* advocating that you stop taking any of your doctor-prescribed medications. That is not the point, so don't be a sheep who follows along blindly. Look, investigate, think, and choose how to take care of your body. Know the score, and make the best decisions for yourself. Then relax and be confident about your choices.

Planting the Seeds of Change

Changing your diet and cutting out junk is really no mystery at all. It's simple: don't buy the junk anymore. Or if you have some, get some heavy-duty garbage bags, go through your cupboards, your refrigerator, and your freezer, and throw away everything unhealthy in a package, box, or can. Don't complain that you spent your hard-earned money to purchase these nonfood items that are hazardous to your health! They're killing you and will eventually cost you more when you become sick and diseased! Throw them out, stare at your empty cupboards, and refrigerator, and wait. Relax, breathe, and smile! When you get hungry enough, real food will look mighty fine!

These days, one in two people dies of heart disease, like my dad did, and one in 2.5 people dies of cancer and the effects of its dangerous treatments, like my mom did. I know now in no uncertain terms that a huge contributor to their early deaths was the way they ate. So if you won't do it for yourself, do you want your kids eating this stuff? What kind of health legacy can they look forward to? Eating junk is a lousy habit, and if you pass it on to your children because you refuse to change, it's a tragedy! Do you really want to leave behind a legacy of disease and misery, all because you were too stubborn to give up your Twinkies and your fettuccine Alfredo?

At some point we all must take responsibility for our health and well-being. All of my sick clients who healed themselves did so because they threw out all the junk in their cupboards. They became educated, took responsibility, took action, and healed and cured themselves. So just do it, and do it today!

What's for Breakfast?

Our digestive juices are most available between 7:00 A.M. and 11:00 A.M. First thing in the morning, however, after a full night's sleep, you are "breaking a fast" (break-fast), so don't bombard your stomach with too much food, too fast. Drink lemon and water upon waking. Thirty minutes later, if you wish, have a single piece of fruit.

Always eat fruits in season and make sure they're organic, but first find out if your body has the capacity to digest fruits. If you've been diagnosed with *Candida albicans*, you'll need to stay away from most fruits until you correct your digestive system, your liver and gallbladder, and rebalance your intestinal flora. Even without *Candida*, if you get gassy and bloated an hour or so after eating any kind of fruit, make other food choices to start your day until you rebalance your body.

Below is a list of fruits I recommend, high in antioxidants, that won't flood your body with too many sugars too fast:

- Berries: all kinds

- Subacid fruits: apples, grapes, peaches, pears, and plums

- Tropical fruits: young (Thai) coconuts, mangoes, papayas, and pineapples

- Acid fruits: grapefruits and oranges

- Melons: melons of all kinds should be eaten alone

- Sweeter fruits: Bananas and sweet fruits should be eaten sparingly, as they tend to cause gas. If you choose to eat them, do so only once or twice a week. Avoid dried fruits altogether unless you reconstitute them—soak them in water all night, which drops the sugar level down.

Remember, it's all about eating balanced and nourishing meals every day to get the broadest possible range of vitamins, macro- and microminerals, amino acids, essential fatty acids, saturated fat, protein, and enzymes in the correct form. That takes preparation, effort, and time that most of us don't have in the morning, so I came up with quick, easy-to-fix solutions that can satisfy your breakfast nutritional needs.

I understand how difficult it is to cut out foods you've been eating for a lifetime. I've often sat across from my very sick clients and seen the look on their faces when I told them they couldn't have their bagel and coffee anymore. They were devastated. "What am I going to eat?" they ask me.

I understood their concern. As I teenager, when I started to educate myself about correct eating, I'd stand in my family kitchen full of junk-food cereals wondering, "What can I eat for breakfast?" After a lot of experimentation, I taught myself how to make nutritious breakfast shakes, and I felt satisfied and energized.

One of the first things I do is teach my patients how to make the same kinds of shakes. To add to the shake, it is advisable to find the broadest base of raw whole food nutrients on the market.

How to Prepare

Put an organic raw food powder into the highest-quality balanced water, or add to raw, sprouted seed, or nut milks.

Add your favorite fruits. Mine are strawberries, blueberries, blackberries, mangoes, coconut juice, and coconut meat (a healthy, unsaturated fat), to name a few.

To the shake add flax and/or borage oil, or sesame oil. As stated previously, add some sort of healthy saturated fat such as raw coconut oil to aid hormone balance and to help create a slow, steady, long-term energy. I believe you can derive as much as two and a half times the energy from a raw-fat molecule as you can from a protein or a carbohydrate molecule. You can also add an avocado.

If you use more than one fruit at a time, you won't get bored with the taste, and each morning's breakfast will be a new experience. Mix, match, and remember to eat foods seasonally. In my shakes, I add banana sparingly because it's high in fruit sugars. And yet a banana can soothe a frazzled nervous system due to its high content of tryptophan, a calming amino acid.

Have you ever tasted young Thai coconuts, with a very thick white husk on the outside and a point at the top? The juice is sweet and delectable, while the meat is soft, delicious, and high in raw, healthy saturated fats and vitamin D. You can add both the juice and the meat to your shake powder and blend it for a superb-tasting treat! Visit my Web site for some of my most popular shake recipes. Find young Thai coconuts in your local health food store or grocery store. Use a cleaver to open the coconut. First, lay the coconut on its side, then carefully bring the cleaver down sharply near the top of the coconut (the pointed side), breaking the inner shell, and immediately set the coconut to rest on its bottom (the flat side) so as not to lose precious coconut water. Drain the coconut water into a glass container, and finish cutting off the top with the cleaver to find the coconut meat. Lift the meat off the shell with the back of a spoon, and remove pieces of shell remaining on the meat. Add the meat to shakes or other recipes.

The following shakes, a few favorites of my clients, family, and friends, are quite beneficial, especially at the beginning of the day. I add different whole foods formulas to these recipes to maximize cellular nutrient intake.

Brantley Basic Thai Coconut Shake

The juice and meat of one Thai coconut

1 cup organic blueberries or strawberries (fresh or frozen)

½ to 1 tsp. lime juice, to taste

1 tbsp. agave syrup, to taste (optional)

Blend ingredients until smooth.

Brantley Tropical Smoothie

Juice of 1 Thai coconut

½ to 1 tsp. of vanilla extract

1 tbsp. bee pollen (optional)

1 tbsp. agave syrup, to taste (optional)

1 pinch cinnamon

2 tbsp. raw, sprouted almond butter for additional protein and thickness (optional)

1 cup mango, papaya, or pineapple, fresh or frozen (choose one only)

½ or whole frozen banana

Blend ingredients until smooth.

Brantley Chocolate Shake

2 cups sprouted nut milk (see recipe on page 158)

1 cup frozen, diced banana

1 to 2 tsp. agave syrup

2 to 3 tbsp. organic cacao nibs or organic cocoa powder

Blend until smooth and creamy.

Brantley Veggie Juice Delight

If you are suffering from an overgrowth of fungus or have blood sugar concerns, start the day with this refreshing vegetable juice. You can add a whole foods formula to it.

Handful organic spinach

1 medium organic cucumber

1 organic tomato

3 stalks organic celery

Juice these organic vegetables and dilute with equal amounts of filtered water.

For Cereal Lovers

For some people, breakfast wouldn't be breakfast without cereal. Your kids may love it, too, but most commercial cereals contain refined sugars or other sweeteners that will quickly elevate blood sugars. They also contain flour and unsprouted grains, additives, artificial colors, preservatives and synthetic vitamins, creating a virtually dead food that can cause physical imbalances and deficiencies. This could set the stage for serious health problems, as your body will view the cereal as a foreign invader, stimulating the white blood cells to mobilize their forces unnecessarily. Now your body is off and running, all because of a few bites of multicolored cereal.

Even if a commercial cereal is labeled "all natural," if the whole grain has not been sprouted and has been ground into flour, it will raise your blood sugar, damaging your insulin levels and putting stress on your immune system. Time and time again, I've observed health food store cereal taxing a client's digestive system, since the unsprouted grains contained enzyme inhibitors. The refined flour and sweeteners released sugars way too quickly, overworking the pancreas, liver, stomach, and intestines.

You need to feed yourself in the morning with an array of nourishing foods so your body can pick and choose the nutrients it needs. If you decide to eat a sprouted cereal, you're doing your body a huge favor. If you are feeling industrious, you can make your own granola or ready-made cereals and use them with the nut milk recipes below.

Brantley'ola Sprouted Nut Cereal

½ cup sunflower seeds, soaked for 2 hours or more

2 cups almonds, soaked overnight

3 cups pecans, soaked overnight

2 cups walnuts, soaked overnight

1 tbsp. vanilla extract

1 tsp. ground cinnamon

Pinch of sea salt to taste

Lightly grind up ingredients in food processor in advance. In the morning, drain water from the nuts and the rest of the ingredients. Refrigerate immediately after the first serving. This will last for two more days. Pour nut milk over the above ingredients. Add agave syrup to taste and add a few of your favorite fruits. My favorites are organic blueberries (fresh or frozen) and fresh organic apple slices.

Brantley No-Time-at-All Nut Milk

1 cup room-temperature filtered water

Pinch of sea salt

½ to 1 tbsp. agave syrup to taste

½ to 1 tsp. of vanilla

Pinch of cinnamon powder (optional)

Pinch of nutmeg (optional)

1 tbsp. organic cocoa or cacao powder (optional)

1 tbsp. raw, sprouted nut butter

Blend until smooth, and refrigerate or use immediately.

Brantley Nut Milk Extra

1 cup raw pecans or 1 cup raw macadamia nuts soaked overnight

3 cups room-temperature filtered water

3 tbsp. agave syrup

1 to 2 tsp. vanilla extract

2 tbsp. coconut butter or 1 tbsp. coconut oil (optional)

Drain the water from the raw pecans or raw macadamias. Blend ingredients until smooth, and refrigerate.

I'm including a few suggestions here to support you in making the transition from your doughnut and coffee to healthier breakfast choices. It's time to stop artificially stimulating your body with sugar and coffee. The sooner you make a commitment to changing your breakfast menus, the sooner your body can heal itself. Nutrition is not about stimulation, it's about nourishment and balance.

Everyone should start the day with a raw-food shake. Because of all the broad-based nutrients it provides, it is the most important part of my program, a must if you want to achieve balance while you maintain and reclaim optimal health.

For those who don't want to give up everything at once, if you crave that piece of toast in the morning, sprouted breads are best, as they contain no enzyme inhibitors to complicate digestion. Sprouted breads are still flour, though, which will have an impact on your blood sugar. Spread raw butter, raw coconut oil, or raw sprouted nut butters on the bread to slow down the release of sugars. To sweeten the toast, use raw, unheated honey or agave syrup, avoiding jams or jellies that contain too much concentrated fruit sugar. Please do not use margarine or any kind of butter substitute, as they contain chemicals not meant for the human body. Toss artificial butters in the trash can, where they belong. Hopefully, sprouted bread or toast will be a transitional food you will eliminate once your habits change.

If you drink more than one cup of coffee a day, you can compensate by increasing your water intake. If you choose to have eggs in the morning, use organic, fertile eggs only. Try to eat them undercooked, and cook them using raw coconut oil or cold pressed virgin olive oil. Add raw vegetables if desired and take plant enzymes before and during the meal.

You can create various fruit bowl combinations for yourself. Go to my Web site (www.Brantleycure.com) for super recipes that I've developed over the years that will knock your socks off!

This is one of my personal favorites.

Brantley Fruit Delight

A handful of each of the following:

Organic blueberries or strawberries (fresh or frozen)

Organic apple pieces, cubed

Organic mango

Pecans or walnuts (soaked and refrigerated from the night before)

1 tbsp. raw coconut oil

½ fresh banana

Pinch of ground cinnamon

Drizzle 1 tbsp. raw coconut oil on top.

Here are some other recipes I've passed on to patients and friends:

Brantley Quick Start Breakfast

1–2 organic oranges, cubed

1 medium avocado, cubed

Handful spouted walnuts or a combination of your favorite nuts (soaked and refrigerated from the night before)

Mix ingredients and enjoy.

Brantley Oatmeal Express

Cooking oatmeal that has been soaked overnight shortens cooking time. (I prefer this oatmeal raw, without cooking.)

Add pecans and walnuts (soaked and refrigerated overnight)

Agave syrup to taste

Pinch of ground cinnamon (optional)

Meat of 1 Thai coconut, chopped

1 tbsp. raw butter or raw coconut oil

Pinch of sea salt

Add favorite nut milk (optional)

Brantley of the Sea Breakfast

Sear salmon or halibut slightly (wild, not farm raised) in small amount of filtered water. After cooking, drizzle cold-pressed virgin olive oil on top. Add garlic powder, cayenne powder, and sea salt to taste. Grate 1 organic carrot and ½ organic beet. Drizzle with cold-pressed virgin olive oil and juice of ¼ organic lemon. Sprinkle salad with sea salt.

For those who have an overgrowth of *Candida albicans* or severe blood sugar challenges, choose foods other than fruit. You can try many different variations of the Brantley of the Sea Breakfast. Or you can add raw cheese to a raw cracker with avocado, tomato, and onion.

Shopping Guide for Breakfast

Whenever possible, use organic meats, fruits and vegetables.

Mix and match the following list of fruits, nuts, and seeds. Be creative. Allow my suggestions to jump-start your imagination to prepare satisfying, nourishing meals.

Fruits: apples, Asian pears, baby (Thai) coconuts, berries, cherries, durians, grapefruits, kiwis, mangoes, oranges, papayas, peaches, pears, plums, pineapples

Nuts and seeds: almonds and raw, sprouted almond butter, flax seeds, macadamia nuts, pecans, sesame and sunflower seeds, walnuts

Vegetables: the sky's the limit!

Don't overwhelm yourself by changing your diet all at once. Concentrate on breakfast alone for two weeks, and don't move ahead until you've made changes. You're setting a new pattern for yourself, and it takes time. When you feel confident and comfortable, let's meet for lunch.

What's for Lunch?

You know how it feels after you've worked all morning. You're really hungry, you have no time, and your work buddies are speeding to the closest, greasiest, and cheapest fast-food joint. Or maybe you can't wait to get to your favorite deli, fantasizing about a smoked turkey and American cheese sandwich on sourdough with chips and a soda.

For many of us, lunch isn't lunch without a sandwich! I know people who've eaten the same sandwich every day of their lives and they never tire of it. If this is you, the bummer is that you may not be tired of your sandwich, but your sandwich is making *you* tired! In fact, a sandwich that contains protein, pasteurized dairy, and refined carbohydrates is one of your greatest enemies.

To make matters worse, many deli meats are high in nitrates, a contributor to stomach cancer, and your digestive organs have to contend with condiments that contain sugar and preservatives, chips fried in partially hydrogenated oil and sprinkled with table salt, and soda loaded with refined sugar, artificial chemicals, and caffeine.

Lunch may be the most challenging meal to change, but don't despair. Let's talk about healthy lunch options.

Whenever possible, use organic meats, fruits, and vegetables.

My suggestion is to take the next week to change your lunch experience. If you can't stand to give up your sandwiches right now, try making the following concessions:

1. You must make your own sandwiches, since I doubt you'll find sprouted bread sandwiches in your local restaurants. Buy sprouted bread, raw cheese, and sliced turkey and chicken from your local health food store, making sure they contain no nitrates or nitrites. Canned tuna in spring water without salt is an okay transition food. Condiments need to be purchased from your local health food store, making sure they contain no canola oil or sugars.

2. If you want to make your own burrito at home, purchase sprouted tortillas. Make sure the beans contain no lard, and stay away from pasteurized cheese. Add guacamole, salsa, and cilantro.

3. For something simple such as vegetables and brown rice, follow my directions below for sprouting grains, seeds and nuts.

How to Sprout and Cook Grains, Seeds, and Nuts

Grains: Add to the grain (millet, brown rice, oatmeal, quinoa, amaranth, etc.) an equal amount of purified, filtered, bottled, or distilled water. Add one tablespoon of raw organic apple cider vinegar or lemon juice (optional). Cover. Let sit at room temperature overnight (seven to ten hours). Drain the water, rinse the grain, and put it back in the pot with an equal amount of purified water. Cook. Cooking time will be shorter for soaked grains.

Seeds and nuts: Put seeds or nuts in a bowl with purified water. If desired, add a pinch of balanced, unrefined sea salt. (Sea salt is optional.) Leave them at room temperature overnight. In the morning, rinse and eat, or rinse and air-dry nuts or seeds on a towel. If you made more than you can eat, dry them and keep refrigerated.

Eat within two or three days. You can rinse these two times a day until consumed. All sprouted breads and tortillas, as well as sliced deli meats such as chicken and turkey, are transitional foods. Sprouted grains are fine.

Optimal Lunch Suggestions

Make sure to take a broad-based plant enzyme twenty minutes before each meal, and take one more during your meal, but if you forget, take them anytime as you eat. If you eat fish or meat, proceed. If not, substitute sprouted nuts, or sprouted seeds, or sprouted legumes (raw cheese is optional). Let these menu suggestions inspire your own creativity.

Brantley Salmon on a String. Lightly seared salmon (as rare as possible in the middle), lightly steamed cabbage and string beans (steam one to three minutes). Add raw butter or cold-pressed olive oil and balanced, unrefined sea salt after steaming. Eat with a large mixed salad.

Brantley Just for the Halibut. Lightly seared halibut or red snapper (as rare as possible in the middle), raw butter and lemon juice after it is seared, salad with diced tomatoes, diced cucumber, chopped parsley, and basil, organic Greek olives, red onions, red pepper sliced thin with olive oil, lemon, or raw organic apple cider vinegar.

Brantley Mermaid Favorite. Sushi-grade tuna sliced raw with a raw vegetable and lettuce salad, olive oil, lemon, and seasonings.

Brantley Chops and Nuts. Raw chopped salad: Choose veggies of all colors. On a plate, arrange grated beets, chopped tomatoes, red peppers, grated carrots, grated yellow squash, chopped cilantro or Italian parsley, and grated purple cabbage. Make an Italian dressing with olive oil, lemon juice, spices, and finely diced parsley and cilantro. Add slices of avocado and sprinkle on top your choice of sprouted sesame seeds, sunflower seeds, almonds, pecans, or walnuts (or any sprouted nut or seed that you prefer).

Brantley Salad of the Sea. Soak arame (or any seaweed you prefer) five to thirty minutes and rinse. Slice the seaweed, green onions, and cucumbers and toss with raw sesame oil and raw apple cider vinegar. Add seasonings, balanced, unrefined sea salt, and sprouted seeds or nuts. Marinate overnight. Eat with steamed corn or steamed yam with raw butter and unrefined sea salt.

Brantley Let Us Rollup. Raw hummus, avocados, tomatoes, and sprouts rolled in lettuce with condiments and spices (add sprouted nuts and seeds if you like). Instead of lettuce, you can substitute nori (a black seaweed), which comes in sheets.

Brantley Let's Get Dicey. Grated carrots, beets, and raw corn with grated jicama and diced cilantro, olive oil, lemon, spices, and unrefined sea salt. If you want to add a protein, feel free. Eat with avocados and raw butter or raw coconut oil on sprouted crackers.

How to Properly Prepare Fish and Meat

Whether you prefer red meat or fish, make sure the meat or the fish is as rare as possible.

Lightly coat the meat in olive oil or raw coconut oil and sear the outside in a pan for two to three minutes, keeping as raw and rare as possible. The healthiest way to prepare fish is to place it on a plate beforehand with herbs. Put the fish with the herbs in a pan with a small amount of water and blanch it, making sure the middle of the fish is as raw as possible. After blanching, remove from the pan and put olive oil or raw butter on top. You can sear in raw oil for a very short time.

Shopping Guide for Lunch

Mix and match the following foods for lunch. Before shopping, if you need more inspiration, please go to my Web site for additional recipes.

Fish: any cold-water fish with scales is okay, wild-caught, not farm-raised, such as salmon, halibut, red snapper, sea bass, tuna.

Meat: grass-fed, hormone-free beef, including hamburger and lamb.

Vegetables: celery, string beans, peas, broccoli, cucumbers, asparagus, all lettuces except iceberg, cauliflower, green and purple cabbage, tomatoes (all colors), Brussels sprouts, sweet potatoes, yams, carrots, beets, summer and winter squash, red-skinned white potatoes, artichokes, avocados, sprouts (any kind), sea vegetables (nori, arame, dulse, hijiki, and kombu), cilantro, parsley, arugula, raw spinach (not cooked), corn, radishes, jicama, peppers (red, yellow, and orange), and many others.

Dairy: raw cheese, raw milk, raw cream, raw butter (nothing pasteurized or homogenized).

Slowly but surely, take the next week to change what you eat for lunch. Remember that you're changing patterns that have been deeply ingrained for a lifetime. Yes, it takes discipline, but you're worth it, so fight for yourself, for your health, and for your life. Don't give it all up for junk food. You have it in you, but you have to give yourself some time. If you can't make these changes in one week, then take longer. Just do as much as you can, don't beat yourself up, and keep drinking your water! Soon, your prior food addictions will quiet down, and your mind will no longer be craving that chocolate bar.

When you start craving a raw vegetable salad or raw cereal, you're on the right track. Remember that you're in the process of unraveling your own so-called health mystery. Isn't it exciting? Just keep going and I'll see you at the dinner table.

What's for Dinner?

By now, you understand and are experiencing the healing power of foods that come from the earth. Your symptoms are probably diminishing, you feel more energy, and you're sleeping through the night. You have an established routine in the morning and at noon, and you are becoming friends with your body.

You have traveled through your day successfully, avoiding those fast-food lunch joints, steering clear of delis and sandwiches. You may have found that great little restaurant close to work that serves healthy food. Or you've figured out what you can bring to work that you already prepared at home. Perhaps you have even had a few comments from your colleagues, saying that you're turning into a health nut. If that's the case, you're definitely heading in the right direction. Pretty soon this new way of eating will be as natural as taking a breath of fresh air.

The following suggestions support healthy choices for dinner. Remember to set the table and let your body pick and choose what nutrients it needs for balance. Eat most of the colors of the rainbow: red, green, yellow, orange, and purple.

Take the next week to ease into these changes for dinner. By now, if you have rehydrated your body and transformed your breakfast and lunch choices, you've cut out enough nonfoods that it will be a snap to utilize my optimal dinner suggestions. As you eat all the nutrients that you need daily—a broad range of vitamins, macro- and microminerals, enzymes, saturated fat, essential fatty acids, and amino acids—your body is rebalancing and renourishing all of your systems. Remember that your body was designed to be a self-correcting, self-healing machine.

Take the next week (or longer) to change your dinner habits. Traditionally, this should be a lighter meal. Don't eat late, and finish your meal at least three hours before bed. If you must eat late at night, make the food as raw as possible. Dinner choices should be simple and easy to digest. If you have a hard time sleeping or unwinding, try a baked potato with steamed veggies, raw butter, or some type of raw oil.

Bon appétit!

Optimal Dinner Suggestions

Whenever possible, use organic meats, fruits, and vegetables.

Brantley Coconut Drizzle. Fruit bowl with fruit of your choice. Drizzle on top raw coconut oil or raw cream. Sprouted nuts or seeds are optional.

Brantley Sear Me Lightly. Lightly seared fish with grated carrots, beets, olive oil, and lemon. Carrots, beets, lemon juice, and olive oil are great to cleanse your liver and gallbladder.

Brantley's Creamy Red Skins. Romaine lettuce, tomato, grated zucchini, raw string beans, lightly steamed red skinned potatoes sliced and tossed with a creamy avocado dressing. In a blender, put avocado, a small amount of water, a little lemon juice, seasonings, and balanced, unrefined sea salt.

Brantley's Beet the Greens. Lightly steamed greens: kale, Swiss chard, collards, and beet greens. Choose one or a combo, and drizzle olive oil or use raw butter and lemon with seasonings.

Brantley's Baked in the Raw. Baked potato with raw butter or olive oil with guacamole and salsa.

Brantley's Corny Salmon. Seared salmon with homemade coleslaw and corn on the cob. Store-bought coleslaw usually has too much mayonnaise and sugar. Chop red and green cabbage, slice some red onion and mix with olive oil, garlic, onion powder, and sea salt, to taste, and fix corn on the cob with raw butter and a pinch of cayenne.

These simple menu suggestions are a jumping-off point. If you splurge on junk food once in a while, enjoy it and don't beat yourself up. After trying these suggested menus for a week and/or branching out on your own, I'm sure you've been faced with eating out in restaurants or attending social gatherings where you wander around in circles, wondering what you can eat for a snack. You go to a party and they have trays of dead food, nonfood, and junk food. And you're hungry! What do you do? I'll teach you how to maneuver any situation and come out feeling great.

Snack Attacks

Now that you have established your personal relationship with breakfast, lunch, and dinner, I'm sure you've achieved a certain amount of personal satisfaction that comes from knowing you are in control. You are no longer being led by the nose, TV commercials don't fool you, and now you know that education is power if you apply it.

What do you do if you miss that healthy meal and you're having a snack attack or craving the crunch? It's three o'clock in the afternoon, you're at work, and you're starving, tired, and stressed. You walk by the coffeepot, you look longingly at the leftover pastries from the morning, you take a few steps toward these delectable goodies—and then you remember: *You are the cause and you are the cure!* Now what?

This can be a huge pitfall for all of us and the feelings of denial can skyrocket sales of chocolate bars! So prepare yourself in advance by bringing raw trail mix and/or raw sprouted food bars to work. If you decide to make a healthier choice, there are a load of so-called protein bars on the market, promising to be low in carbohydrates, fats, and sugars. They aren't healthy. What they are is a glorified, healthy-sounding candy bar.

If you want to get some snack bars, everything in that bar needs to be alive, healthy, and raw. There are a few healthy, raw bars available, but make sure you read labels. Even if the bar is raw, it can still be too high in sugars. "But what about the crunch?" you ask yourself, one of the biggest complaints I get from clients. "If I can't have my tortilla chips," they bargain, "then you sure as heck better replace them with something that satisfies my need for the crunch!"

In the past couple of years, numerous companies have come out with raw and dehydrated crackers and chips tasting mostly like sawdust. The crunch treats I suggest should be balanced, living snacks stacked with nutrients. You need to find raw sprouted crackers that taste great. Visit my Web site for raw bar and raw cracker suggestions.

If a snack leaves you craving another sweet goodie, your body is most likely deficient in raw fat and raw protein. In this case, I advise my clients to eat half a teaspoon of raw coconut oil or half a teaspoon of raw butter if they're still craving the candy bar. Put it on a raw sprouted cracker if you wish. It tastes terrific, and you'll be surprised at how fast your sugar cravings disappear.

Other Brantley Snack suggestions:

> Apples, walnuts, pecans, or almonds
>
> Sprouted trail mix
>
> Celery sticks with raw, sprouted almond or cashew butter
>
> Guacamole with sliced cucumber, carrots, and red bell pepper strips
>
> Sprouted crackers with fresh salsa

Once again, it's all about balance and being able to figure out what your body is trying to tell you.

Restaurants

It's hard to imagine that you can actually eat well if you are not at a health food café. That is not always the case. When you go out to eat at a restaurant, start out by sending the bread basket away before it hits the table. Then think about the guidelines for breakfast, lunch, and dinner. Better yet, before you even go out anywhere, make sure you eat a healthy snack so you don't grab the first thing that comes your way. If you're already hungry before you even leave the house, take a moment and make a raw-food shake.

Proper food combining is a very important key, which means no protein and carbohydrates at the same meal, and fruit should be eaten alone. Meat and potatoes or meat and rice (even brown rice) are out. Think simple and fresh. You can always get a salad dressed with olive oil and lemon, and you can bring sea salt with you, since commercial dressings are filled with sugar and preservatives.

Order your fish seared, leaving the middle raw, and ask them not to use table salt or oil. You can put on olive oil (cold-pressed) after it is seared, when it comes to the table. With red meat, ask them to sear it quickly on both sides, using no oil. Either way, the available protein choices are not likely to be organic, so you may want to order a salad or potato and steamed veggies instead. That's up to you.

Dessert, my friends, is not an option. Remember, it's digestive suicide to eat any sugary dessert immediately after a meal, especially after a meal with animal protein. The more you are feeding yourself what your body needs for balance, the less you will crave desserts after a meal. If there are beautiful fruit choices right after the meal, take enzymes. Don't order ice cream, sauce, or whipped cream to eat with the fruit. Mother Nature's garden needs no improvements.

Dinner Parties

When you're sitting down at someone's dining room table, staring at pizza and spaghetti with marinara sauce, it's a challenge to figure out what to do. I've found, more often than not, that the host or hostess will offer salad. I heap it on my plate and enjoy it immensely, making sure the host knows it was the best salad I ever ate. That lessens her upset when it's the only thing I eat, and she doesn't feel that I'm judging how they choose to eat.

I simply refuse to compromise my health to make other people feel comfortable by eating their nonfood. It they try to talk me into eating that plate of pasta, for example, I laugh and change the subject. The point here is that you can keep on track in any eating situation without drawing too much attention to yourself. There is always a carrot or celery stick somewhere. In fact, my friends always say that I could find something healthy to eat in the middle of the Mojave Desert, and I have no doubt that they're right.

How about that gooey, chocolaty birthday cake when your best friend is turning fifty? There is no law declaring it essential that you indulge. Who made that rule up? Wishing your friend a hearty happy birthday and protecting your body from an onslaught of refined sugar are perfectly appropriate in my book. In fact, it's pretty darned smart! I know the cake looks great, but nothing is worth the damage it will do to your system. You've worked too hard to cave in to the temptation and the pressure.

In fact, those gooey, chocolaty, cheesy, sugary desserts look disgusting to me now, which is the result of eating for balance. But if you do slip back and dive into the chocolate birthday cake, don't beat yourself up. Everyone will cheat once in a while. Make sure you take a good plant enzyme and an herbal detoxification product when you get home. This should rescue you from any damage.

If you are standing in front of a big buffet, walk past the bread, pasta and pasta salad, desserts, chips, cheese, and crackers, and anything gooey that looks like it's been prepared with a pound of hydrogenated fat. Look for the fish, the meat, the cooked veggies (hopefully without sauce), and the raw veggies. Then fill your plate before you have a chance to dip into the dip! I fill my plate with veggies for dipping and have a great meal when there are no other food choices.

One last reminder: Before you go to a questionable food function, feed yourself beautifully with something like a live raw-food shake with extra oils. This should fill you up so well that you can happily and politely nibble veggies for the rest of the night.

Please remember that snacks, eating out, and parties are not an excuse to eat forbidden nonfood. Your body doesn't care what you're celebrating or who wants you to eat cake and ice cream. Your body is busy doing its job, trying to keep you balanced and alive. Don't make it harder. Stay conscious and don't say, "Ah, what the heck. I'll eat only one handful of chips." Just keep feeding your body naturally, always asking yourself, *Will my actions tonight hurt my body or heal it?*

Don't be afraid to set yourself apart from unhealthy people and habits. Instead, enjoy the foods that come directly from the land and the sea. Eat right, drink right, and you will be merry!

There are options, so let's start with my complete list of so-called foods to avoid. I wanted to make it easy for you, so you don't have to guess what to throw out or avoid. I created this list after working with thousands of patients over many years who shared with me their lifestyle patterns of eating and drinking. Based on my work with them, we discovered that what they had consumed greatly contributed to the cause of their health problems. Feel free to place this list on your refrigerator, prop it up on your desk at work, or place it in your wallet or purse, since it could save your life.

For Optimal Health, *do not* eat the following nonfoods:

1. Pasta or pizza

2. Refined or whole grain breads

3. Flour products, including muffins, scones, Danish pastries, bagels, doughnuts, Pop-Tarts, cinnamon rolls, and white or wheat toast or buns

4. Processed or refined flour crackers or tortilla chips of any kind, including Doritos, Goldfish, Triscuits, potato chips, Frito-Lays, saltines, and Wheat Thins

5. Rice cakes

6. Commercial cereals

7. Table salt

8. Tortillas (wheat or corn)

9. Sugar or artificial sweeteners such as Aspartame (Nutrasweet) and Splenda (Sucralose)

10. Pasteurized dairy foods of any kind, including pasteurized milk, cheese, cream cheese, sour cream, and cottage cheese

11. Hot dogs; deli meats containing nitrates or nitrites, including turkey, ham, beef, pastrami, salami, pepperoni, and corned beef; smoked meats are dangerous to the lining of your stomach

12. Bacon, including Canadian bacon

13. Canned fruits and vegetables

14. Processed and packaged foods

15. Frozen meals and frozen processed foods

16. Sugar, candy, ice cream, cookies, pies, cakes, and cupcakes

17. Fast food, including Taco Bell, Arby's, McDonald's, Carl's Junior, Burger King, In and Out Burger, fast-food pizza joints,

fast-food Chinese, Subway, KFC, Popeye's Chicken, and any other fast-food restaurants

18. Fried foods, such as French fries, onion rings, fried chicken or chicken wings, and fried zucchini sticks

19. Popcorn with fake butter flavor

20. Condiments with sugar, table salt, or preservatives; that includes sugary ketchup and mayonnaise

21. Preservatives, additives, and hydrogenated or partially hydrogenated oils; read the labels before buying anything, even if you think you know all the ingredients; if you can't pronounce it or you can't identify it, don't buy it!

22. Caffeine and caffeinated teas

23. Bottled or packaged fruit and vegetable juices

24. Margarine or butter substitutes of any kind, including lard, shortening, and processed vegetable oil

Now that you've read this list, you're probably panicking and wondering what you can eat. Read on for inspiration that will lead you into the world of good eating and good health.

The Land of Fruits and Vegetables

Proceed to the produce section of your health food store. Look around. This, my friends, is real food that comes from the earth. Isn't it beautiful? There are aisles and aisles of real food in this section of the store, and you get to buy anything you like. Go crazy! Pick and choose your favorite real foods and pile them in your cart. Organic produce is always preferred, but if you don't live near a farmer's market or health food store, you can buy a fruit and vegetable wash at your local grocery store to wash off the pesticides.

Always remember that junk food, processed and packaged food, and foods that glow in the dark are not meant for human consumption! Just think, if you've lived primarily on junk food for most of your life, and real food has rarely passed your lips, maybe that's why you're sick and suffering.

When someone tells me that if they can't eat junk food, there's nothing to eat, I recall starving people who would fall down and weep if they walked into a produce department and saw the beautiful fruits and vegetables there for the buying. If you always shop on the perimeter of the grocery store where you will find the produce and meat, you will always be filled with nature's foods. If the only things you like in the produce section are iceberg lettuce and red Delicious apples, it's time to expand your horizons. If you want to turn your life around and live well, you'll have to become intimate friends with the extensive fruit and vegetable kingdom. You have no choice, because you *cannot* get healthy on iceberg lettuce and ranch dressing!

Try introducing two or three new fruits and vegetables into your diet every couple of weeks, until they become new members of your family. Then get creative and try other fruits and vegetables. Give your palate time to readjust. It will take patience and compliance, but when you start to clear out some of those toxins in your body, you'll stop craving junk food as real food choices will start to taste better.

Meats and Fish

If you eat meat and fish, proceed to those sections. If your market does not have fresh fish wild-caught, not farm-raised, and if the meat is not organic and hormone-free, walk out! There is a pesticide wash to rid produce of chemicals, but nothing can clean hormones or chemicals out of the flesh of meat and fish.

If your market sells fresh fish and organic, hormone-free meat, consider the wide range of possibilities. Remember, you don't have to fry or stir-fry it, bread or barbecue it, stew it, skewer or pressure-cook it to make it taste delicious. Make it simple by eating organic meat or fish as rare as possible, always heading toward eating as raw as you can. You can lightly blanch with water and herbs or sear with raw oil and herbs. Just keep it simple.

Raw Cold-Pressed Oils

The healthiest raw oils are usually offered online or in a health food store. Supermarkets are way behind the times when it comes to anything that supports optimal health. If you never cook, hate to cook, or don't know how, then you're in the perfect position to eat raw—the way we were intended to eat!

Balanced, Unrefined Sea Salt

Using unrefined sea salt is one of the most important aspects of regaining and maintaining your health. Finding this salt, however, was one of my greatest challenges, because although there are many salts on the shelf, most are refined, which means they are dangerous to your health. Even some of the ones that say "natural sea salt" are usually refined, and therefore not balanced, so beware. With balanced salts, you probably won't experience the same negative side effects of table salt, such as thirst, dehydration, or swelling of the hands and feet. How wonderful to use these unrefined salts with none of the side effects that we suffer when using refined table salt.

CHAPTER 15

Taking Out the Garbage

Intestinal Detox

You have no idea what a celebration your tissues, organs, blood, and glands are having as a result of your new eating habits. You may not have noticed, but you have called the movers, you are changing your address, and you are slowly moving out of the garbage dump. Now it's time to have the movers haul the old garbage out. Then and only then can your body achieve optimal health.

Let's face it. Who can tolerate the smell of raw sewage? What makes us think that the garbage that lies putrefying inside of us doesn't smell the same? If you take out the garbage, your home doesn't smell. If you don't, it stinks to high heaven. This is taking place right now inside your body. You are feeding it the good stuff, but the old undigested stuff is still stuck there. Why do you think pasta sticks to the wall? People are literally gluing their intestines shut!

If you still think your intestines don't need a thorough cleansing, listen to this: a clogged or dirty intestinal tract can cause any number of problems elsewhere in the body. Dr. Norman Walker tells an amazing story about a young woman and her parents who came to see him. She

175

was in her early twenties and had been suffering from severe epilepsy since she was thirteen. After reviewing X-rays of her colon (her parents found that unusual), Dr. Walker diagnosed distention and distortion in her colon and said she needed to do a series of colonics. He also advised this woman to drink raw juices and eat a diet of raw foods. Suspecting that her bowel toxicity was contributing to her condition, he told her she probably had parasites.

When advised that she get colonics six days a week for five to six weeks and remain strictly on his suggested eating protocol, she reluctantly agreed, but really had no idea what her colon had to do with her epilepsy. After all, wasn't it about her brain and her electrical system? Her parents thought this suggested treatment sounded absurd, but they agreed because they didn't know what else to do.

Three weeks went by and nothing out of the ordinary was revealed in the glass tube during the daily hour of her colon irrigations. She was discouraged, and her parents were feeling like they were wasting their money on this ridiculous treatment, but Dr. Walker convinced them to finish the course of treatment, and they agreed.

At the end of the fifth week, she suddenly sat straight up on the colonic table and passed a large amount of toxic sludge. After that, she finished the six weeks of raw juices, raw foods, and colonics, and her epileptic seizures disappeared, never to come back. So even if you think your problems have nothing to do with toxic buildup in your bowel, you may be wrong.

Now that you're hydrated and your diet is relatively clean, keep in mind that you can't cleanse your intestines with a Coke in one hand and an enema tube in the other! The first step is to start drinking freshly squeezed vegetable juices every day, morning and evening.

Upon waking, drink eight ounces of hot water with the juice from ¼ of an organic lemon. For most intestinal problems such as constipation, colitis, gastritis, or a toxic bowel, I suggest a juice combination of carrot and spinach to encourage your intestines to clear out. This combination will also refurbish your intestines and clear some space for a thorough intestinal cleansing.

Start with eight ounces of freshly squeezed juice (drink immediately upon juicing) and increase your daily amount for a week until you're up to a minimum of sixteen ounces to thirty-two ounces per day. Cut your fresh juice with water. If you have blood sugar issues and you feel tired after drinking this juice combination, lower the amount of carrot juice, which is high in natural sugars.

Years ago, when I was faced with how to cleanse my toxic intestines, there were very few intestinal detoxification products from which to choose. Today there is a wide range of detox products. Do your homework.

First, find a formula that starts to clear the waste and toxins out of the entire body. As that waste starts to move out, your sluggish bowels should start to respond over the next week or so. This first step is very important. You should have at least two bowel movements per day, if not more. Give your body time to adjust. A slow removal of the toxins is much better than dumping years of toxins into your bloodstream.

When your bowels are moving every day, you can then add a herbal formula that softens the hardened mucoid plaque on the inside walls of the small and large intestines. This formula will also act like a broom, removing the years of accumulated waste material, greatly increasing the amount of stool that is passed. If your intestines are impacted with toxins and sludge, a simple castor oil pack applied to the abdomen for thirty minutes each night can help break up stagnated waste material. Use a good-quality castor oil (from the castor bean, not the motor oil; it's been used effectively for thousands of years) without additives or preservatives and saturate a piece of white, washed flannel, large enough to cover your abdomen. Place the saturated flannel across your abdomen, then cover with plastic wrap and an old towel. Place a heating pad on top of the towel and sit or lie down quietly for thirty minutes. Discard flannel and take a shower. If you have difficulty washing the castor oil from your skin, put baking soda on a wet washcloth, rub gently, and rinse.

If you want a deeper cleansing of your intestinal tract, consider fasting as you take the herbal formulas. This has to be your call. If you can handle fasting, for the first cleanse, fast no more than two to three days. Fasting during this cleansing period will encourage your body to shed toxins faster. If you have headaches, body aches, or fatigue, this most likely means that you are detoxifying. However, if these symptoms are too overwhelming, give yourself a few days off, then resume when your symptoms subside. If your detoxification symptoms continue to plague you, at the end of each day run a comfortable hot bath to cover your entire body. Add 1 cup Epsom salts and soak for approximately twenty to thirty minutes. Continue to add hot water when it starts to cool. After soaking, rinse in the shower. This will draw toxins out through your pores.

On alternate days, take a baking soda bath. It helps to alkalize an acidic system, leaving you feeling calm and refreshed. Fill the bath with comfortably hot water, submerge your body, and dissolve 8 ounces of baking soda into the water. Soak for twenty to thirty minutes and rinse in shower. Then, immediately wrap yourself in a towel and lie down for at least twenty minutes.

Just remember that when you do cleanse, adequate rest is vitally important. Be in bed no later than 10:00 P.M.—this is not the time to burn the candle at both ends. Your body needs a chance to do its work. Can you afford dipping into your reserve energy to clean house? Your body naturally goes into a cleansing cycle at night. Make sure you finish your last meal at least three hours before bed, so if you work late, bring something you can eat in the early evening to maintain your natural rhythm.

You will need patience with this process. Some people may be ready to start shedding those layers of unwanted toxins right away. Others may need repeated cleanses over time to achieve the same results. Eventually, though, if you fast and cleanse, you'll see strings of thin, rubbery mucus or hardened, thicker layers passing, in the form and shape of the inside of your intestinal walls. As usual, the color and texture will vary from person to person, depending on eating history and present health and constitution.

For each day you fast, wait a week before cleansing again. For example, if you fasted during your cleanse for three days, wait three weeks to repeat your cleanse. If you fasted for seven days, then wait seven weeks before repeating the cleanse.

Once you have done the deep cleansing for however many months you deem necessary, you need to make sure to repeat this cleanse at least two to three times a year—for life. Like cleaning your house and the outside of your body, the name of the game is *clean it up and keep it clean*. Your body will be grateful.

Now let's move to the next step in your detoxification process: the liver and the gallbladder.

Liver/Gallbladder Detox

The liver is on call twenty-four hours a day and has many difficult tasks to accomplish to ensure your survival. The liver's main job is to clean your blood, nonstop. It filters, neutralizes, and eliminates anything you've eaten, inhaled, or absorbed that could be toxic to your body. It constantly attempts to trap all pharmaceutical drugs, undigested food particles, viruses, bacteria, fungi, dead cells, debris, alcohol, household cleaners, perfumes, dyes, preservatives, and additives. Add to the list personal-care items that have been absorbed through your skin such as hair spray, deodorant, creams, soap residue, makeup, man-made toxins, pesticides, and everything that is manipulated, turned into a chemical, and processed.

Perhaps you've noticed that you can't eat fatty foods any more. That's because your liver and particularly your gallbladder are clogged. One of the gallbladder's functions is to store bile, a waste product of the liver that contains neutralized poisons. But bile also stimulates digestion, ensuring the proper breakdown of fats and stimulating peristalsis, the rhythmic waves of the large intestine to induce a bowel movement. Since the liver and the gallbladder are essential for proper digestion and good health, if they are failing, so are you! Every client I've ever seen has felt much better after cleaning his or her liver and gallbladder. In my opinion, everyone needs to do this.

During this cleansing process, you must continue to make sure your elimination organs keep moving out the toxins. You don't want toxins leaving your liver and racing to your intestines and kidneys, where they must compete for exit space. It's like screaming "Fire!" in a crowded movie theater—if everyone goes for the same exit, it's chaos. Likewise, if the toxins can't get out fast enough, they recirculate in the blood, your lymph glands get overloaded, the toxins flow back into your blood, and they get deposited somewhere else in your body. Not good!

Find powerful herbal formulas that effectively clean out your liver and gallbladder. For your liver, you need an herbal formula that will soften and eliminate the years of hardened toxins. This formula should also contain herbs that can renourish your liver. For your gallbladder, you need to find an herbal formula that will slowly soften and dissolve the gallstones and hardened cholesterol molecules into liquid for easy elimination.

If you have gallstones and are in pain or discomfort, try taking the following:

Raw apple juice. Eight ounces of organic raw apple juice will generally calm symptoms. Don't use any apple juice in a bottle from a store shelf. You won't get the same benefits. Fresh-squeezed apple juice helps to reduce inflammation, but if you have blood sugar issues, cut the fresh apple juice with pure water. I suggest using Granny Smith apples; they are less sweet than others and therefore have been well tolerated by most of my blood-sugar-sensitive clients.

The Daily Program

I believe in preparing the body in advance, slowly easing into the liver/gallbladder flush instead of shocking it with a big flush without preparation. If you've been diagnosed with gallstones, proceed with caution. You need to prepare your liver and gallbladder for at least five if not seven days before you do the flush. If you've done a flush before, you may choose to prepare for only three days. You be the judge. Prepare as follows:

Daily Drink. Mix the following ingredients in a blender and drink all day, every day before the big flush:

  1 oz. organic lemon juice

  1 oz. organic lime juice

  14 oz. organic orange juice

  16 oz. pure or distilled water

  1 slice of fresh ginger

  1 clove of garlic (optional but will improve results)

If desired, use raw apple juice instead of lemon, lime, and orange juice. Raw apple juice can cause bloating, as it is high in natural sugars, so choose whatever seems appropriate for your body.

Add an herbal gallstone dissolver to the daily drink. It will slowly soften and emulsify the stones and years of accumulated hardenings in the gallbladder. It also will help to cleanse the liver.

Water intake. Drink up to 50 percent of your body weight in ounces of pure water. For example, if you weigh 180 pounds, you should drink 90 ounces of pure water.

Food intake. Eat simply, such as fresh fruit in the morning and organic raw vegetable salads in afternoon and evening. Stay away from all cooked foods.

Every evening. At six o'clock, take a liver/gallbladder herbal detoxifier. At nine o'clock, stir or blend one ounce of cold-pressed virgin olive oil and one ounce of grapefruit juice. Drink immediately.

Repeat this protocol each day. This lead-up protocol prepares your liver and gallbladder for the final flush, slowly and gently softening your clogged and hardened organs as well as any stones you may have. The length of the lead-up time is up to you, but you *must* do it for at least three days before the flush. You need to give your body time to unlayer all that muck from your liver and gallbladder.

The Day of the Liver/Gallbladder Flush

Depending on how long you have prepared, on the last day, if you're still eating, fast after breakfast for the rest of the day. Some people find it more effective to fast for two to three days before the final flush.

Continue the daily drink with a herbal gallstone-dissolving formula.

6:00 P.M.: take a herbal detoxifier

9:00 P.M.: blend the following ingredients thoroughly and drink quickly:

4 to 6 oz. cold-pressed virgin olive oil

6 oz. fresh organic grapefruit juice

juice of one organic lemon

Immediately after chugging the flush drink, lie in a fetal position on your right side with a hot-water bottle over your liver/gallbladder area (under the ribs on your right side) for thirty minutes.

What to Expect

After drinking the flush drink, you may feel nauseated. A few people may vomit. This doesn't happen often, but it's a perfectly normal indication that your liver and gallbladder are very clogged. If you vomit, your flush will still produce results.

Try to be patient, since it usually takes some hours for your bowels to open up. During the flush, bowel movements are extremely loose and soft. If you want to see what comes out, gallstones look like green peas in your feces. There also may be hardened yellow, green, or white chunks, among other things. If you don't see anything, don't worry. Your toxins and stones may already have been thoroughly emulsified and eliminated. Be aware that the first time you do a liver/gallbladder flush, the toxic smell is unbelievable! This is an example of all that has been clogged in there for years.

The day after the flush, the liver, gallbladder, and large intestine usually purge on and off until mid- to late morning. If your gallbladder is very clogged, you may have very uncomfortable symptoms until your gallbladder softens and releases, so be patient. After that, your appetite will most likely return. Please eat lightly and wisely the rest of the day, drinking distilled or purified water with fresh lemon. Rest. At night, keep the toxins moving by taking a full-body herbal detoxifier.

Your liver and gallbladder will continue to dump toxins well after you finish your flush, so don't be surprised if you feel fatigued for a few days. Your body uses a lot of energy to purge those toxins, but it is energy well spent. If you see no gallstones eliminating, don't get discouraged. Your liver and gallbladder will slowly soften over time, and soon enough, those gallstones will come out, if you have them. Even if you don't have them, you'll still be cleaning out years of toxins. If you have continued discomfort in your liver or gallbladder, you can repeat this flush in three weeks. For optimal health, do at least two of these extended flushes per year.

Now let's continue on our campaign to clean up the highways and byways of your body. It's time for a kidney/bladder detox

Kidney/Bladder Detox

If you don't have kidney stones, kidney disease, or chronic bladder infections, it doesn't mean that your kidneys are functioning at 100 percent capacity. If you've ever eaten junk food in your life, your kidneys are probably partially clogged, not working efficiently.

We live in an imperfect world. We breathe dirty air, we eat dirty food, we drink dirty liquids, and it all must be eliminated through the intestines, kidneys, or skin. If you don't clean them, your body's balance will suffer, and if one organ is affected, so are all the others, because they work as a team. If you clean your intestines and/or your liver and gallbladder but forget your poor overworked kidneys, you are defeating the purpose.

Let's attend to our important filters—our kidneys.

Watermelon. This is brilliant for cleaning out the kidneys and the blood, a great way to get things rolling before a kidney/bladder detox. Eating watermelon in the summer is cooling, refreshing, and satisfying, and it will help your body move toxins out fast.

The watermelon fast. Eat nothing but watermelon for two to three days. No other food or juices. Make sure to drink water as well.

To come off the watermelon fast. Do this slowly with another piece of fruit. Then eat a raw salad. Wait a couple of days to eat nuts, seeds, or more concentrated foods.

Kidney/Bladder Flush Program

Follow this flush for seven days.

You will need a very comprehensive but gentle herbal combination to cleanse your kidneys and your bladder. Many times, our kidneys and/or bladder are filled with toxins, infection, or inflammation without our ever experiencing symptoms. It is imperative to find the perfect herbal combination for this flush.

Once again, it is very important to find a product that can efficiently dissolve both kidney stones and bladder calculus. It is not any easy task to find such a product, but it is vitally important for the purposes of this flush.

Food intake. Eat simply, using raw fruits and vegetables. No cooked food while on the program, especially meat protein, as it taxes the kidneys.

Fasting. This is optional for a deeper cleanse. It will give your kidneys a rest from the hard work of trying to eliminate toxins from both digested and undigested food and drink. Fast on celery, parsley, and carrot juices, using only a small amount of carrot juice.

For optimal products for each of these cleanses, see the resource section at the back of this book. You also can visit my Web site at www.Brantleycure.com for various other cleansing options.

CHAPTER 16

Sun, Spirit, Exercise, Rest, Relaxation, Fun, and Forgiveness

Now that your body is becoming balanced (a major accomplishment!), it's time to address other things that will bring balance into your everyday life. I call this chapter "SSERRFF"—Sun, Spirit, Exercise, Rest, Relaxation, Fun, and Forgiveness.

Sun. Sunlight, one of the most crucial elements for overall health, has been sorely misrepresented by the modern medical industry. A small amount of sunlight on your skin (twenty to thirty minutes a day) is vital for the production of vitamin D_3 (cholecalciferol), and essential for the absorption of calcium and other minerals. The sun's UVB rays react with cholesterol both inside and on the surface of the skin, creating vitamin D_3, which helps you absorb and utilize calcium.

Vitamin D_3 ensures that our cellular nutrition goes through the proper cycle of metabolism, and the calcium ion, which opens the door to deliver the nutrients to the cell, depends on vitamin D_3. A balanced diet rich in omega-3 essential fatty acids (from fish or flax oil) also will give you vitamin D_3. If you don't live in the sun belt or high in the mountains where UBV rays are more potent, you might want to consider taking cod-liver oil, which contains naturally occurring vitamin D_3. After the summer months, you can derive naturally occurring vitamin D_3 from organ meats, eggs, and fish. Do *not* supplement with synthetic vitamin D_2 (ergocalciferol).

Did you know that in primitive cultures around the world where they eat directly from the earth and the sea, they have very few problems with skin cancer or melanoma? Centenarians around the world expose their entire body to a full spectrum of sunlight daily, so watch your diet, and have fun in the sun; just don't stay out too long.

Spirit. It's up to each of us to keep our spirits positive and alive. I advise you to watch your self-talk, since undeniable statistics indicate that what we tell ourselves determines our experience. Are you saying nice things about yourself and others, or are you constantly berating yourself and criticizing others? Now that you're eating and drinking well, it's time to change your attitude about healing, aware that whatever symptoms have plagued you can and will change. Remind yourself that God made our bodies with self-healing abilities and that divine health is your birthright.

It helps others when we build hearts of compassion and renew our spirits, taking the attention off ourselves and onto someone else in need. The act of giving to another physically releases endorphins (well-being hormones) in you and your loved one. No matter your religion or what you believe, daily prayers and good wishes for yourself and others can connect you to the deepest love and healing in the world.

Exercise. Our bodies are meant to be active every day, as we encourage our muscles to tear down and rebuild with added strength. When we exercise, we promote circulation and we pull in oxygen, which is important to fight cancer, viruses, bacteria, fungi, and other potential destroyers that can't live in a highly oxygenated body. As I mentioned, a short time on a minitrampoline will help wash away trapped fluids around the cells and remove toxins while increasing the electrical potential of each cell as well as communication between cells.

Low-impact exercise is the safest and the least stressful to your joints, so choose what you like, whether it's walking, swimming, or riding a bike. By the way, the walk to the kitchen for a bag of chips and then back to the couch to watch TV is not what I call exercise.

Exercising your mind by reading a good book and learning something new is also extremely important to your overall health. Challenge yourself by getting some life back into that oxygen-starved mind and body. Move forward and celebrate your life. Wake up and smell the roses—at least five blocks down the street!

Rest and Relaxation. God created the world in six days, so the Bible says, and on the seventh day, He rested. If rest is good enough for God, do you think it might be good enough for you? I cannot stress how crucial rest and adequate sleep are to your restoration. The old adage "Early to bed and early to rise makes a man healthy, wealthy, and wise," goes along with the natural circadian rhythm of our bodies, which follows the cycle of the sun and the moon.

We were designed to sleep when the sun sets, to wake when the sun rises, and to eat a healthy diet in between. No matter how much we groan and gnash our teeth, that is how the body was designed, and straying from that rhythm will cause the immune system to suffer. After the sun goes down, it is time for the body to slow down so it can rest and repair. If we eat late at night, our body must use its energy to digest when it should be in a rest-and-rebuild cycle. If any of our energy is to be used at all, it should be used for regenerating, not digesting. Moonlight affects the pituitary gland, which is important to hormone production and the ruler of our endocrine system, and a lack of pituitary nourishment will cause all of our organs to suffer.

Even for confirmed night owls, the balance of your body is at stake if you violate these principles. In Chinese medicine, you protect your postnatal jing (metabolic reserve) by thinking, eating, and sleeping well. We can't expect this miraculous body of ours to support a crazy and exhausting lifestyle filled with late-night drugging, partying, and bad eating. If you stress out by overworking your adrenal glands until you are exhausted, you will force your cortisol (stress hormone) levels through the roof, turning your body acid, forcing oxygen out, and inviting illness in.

When animals are tired, they sleep. All living creatures need rest. If we don't allow the soil to rest, replenish, and regenerate, it becomes what we call tired soil, depleted of its mineral content, causing terrible deficiencies in our diets if food grown in this soil is eaten. I even encourage my clients who are not critically ill to take a rest from all supplements and herbal formulas one day a week. Personally, I fast for twenty-four hours once a week. Each night before sleep, in the middle of the night, and first thing in the morning, I talk to God, to rest my soul and renourish my spirit.

Fun. Most of us work too hard and play too little. Remember how it felt to play like a child? Don't you miss hanging around with family and friends, acting silly and carefree? It's time to have some fun, such as taking off your shoes and walking barefoot on the grass. We all need to have fun and fly high on a natural endorphin release. It is so beneficial for body, mind, and soul.

Forgiveness. No matter how horrible your circumstances, a lack of forgiveness will hurt you in the end, as the hate festers and could contribute to giving you cancer or heart disease. Health is also about your mind and the feelings you carry in your heart. As odd as it may sound, I have witnessed that an unwillingness to forgive can cause an acidic condition in the body, forcing oxygen out of the cells and stagnating the body's energy. Scientific studies on the power of forgiveness have proven this to be more than a fictional concept, so if you can't forgive someone in person, try writing your feelings in a journal so you can let them go.

We all make mistakes, no one is perfect, and I'm grateful my father taught me never to go to bed angry or bitter. At an early age, I learned the value of loving, hugging, and showing affection and appreciation to loved ones. After all, we never know how long we will be on this earth.

"Never go to bed with regrets," my dad said. "Clean the slate with God. Say you're sorry before you turn out the lights, and you'll sleep like a baby."

He was right. It is only by nourishing ourselves with the best food, drink, and thoughts that we can truly be free from suffering, pain, and negativity.

CHAPTER 17

The Obesity Cure

The answer to obesity is not finding the right diet. It's about finding balance! Many of you who are trying to lose weight have done everything imaginable but sew your mouth shut! Most times, even if you *have* lost weight, food addictions—physical or emotional—are so strong, it's nearly impossible to keep the weight off for long. We eat to fill up our empty existence, to fit in, or to press down painful emotions.

We all know how it feels to shove food into our mouths when we're not even hungry, eating enormous quantities before our poor stomach has a chance to signal that it's already full. If we actually manage to lose some weight on a fad diet, we end up starved for nutrition, inadvertently flooding our systems with toxins that have previously been stored in our fatty tissue. As our toxic level rises, our cravings return and we eat those non-foods all over again, only to return to a lifetime pattern of yo-yo dieting. Once we eat those forbidden foods again, our weight spirals and we're left demoralized, sinking deeper into the land of rationalization and self-hatred.

If you're still asking why you haven't been able to conquer the battle of the bulge, you're not listening to the most basic principle: *it's all about balance*. If your body is carrying excess toxins and poisons, some of which are stored in the fat tissues, your body is never free to do its job. When you change your diet and stop eating junk, your body no longer needs to use energy to convert the excess sugar to fat. If you're not taking in an overabundance of nonfoods, your body can burn the excess fat you've already stored.

To gain victory over the waddle, you need to begin by detoxifying your intestines, thereby preventing the excess waste from being stored in the body. By detoxifying your liver and gallbladder, you can remove hardened cholesterol molecules, freeing your liver and gallbladder to break down and utilize the excess fat for energy. When the gallbladder is cleared of gallstones, it can more efficiently release bile salts to break down the raw fats you are now including in your meals, which will be converted to energy, not fat. The good news is that if you're eating correctly, raw fats will not be your enemy.

Obviously, you need to exercise as well. If you are overweight, try building up slowly to thirty minutes of cardio, five days a week. It will kick up your metabolism and help you burn excess fats. Time and time again, when my clients started nourishing and cleansing properly, the weight just fell off, even when they weren't coming to me to lose weight. That was the least of their problems, since they were seriously ill, but adherence to my philosophy led to restoration and balance, while unwanted poundage disappeared—along with the associated risks of diabetes, heart disease, and cancer.

Don't forget that it's all about balance. It's not about starving yourself or going on a water fast or jogging five miles wrapped in Saran Wrap to sweat off the pounds. Who can keep any of that up? Diets don't work! As a matter of fact, they cause imbalances. Don't concentrate on your weight. You are done with that! If you are doing the right things, eventually your body will balance itself out and your health will be restored.

Madeline Hammond's Story

There is no greater example of this than Madeline Hammond, associate publisher of *Variety* magazine. She was fifty pounds overweight when I met her on April 2, 1999. She was depressed and suffering from severe allergies. Her test results revealed a low immune response, parasites, an imbalanced GI tract, yeast and uric acid crystals, vitamin and mineral deficiencies, a hormonal imbalance, a toxic liver, a histamine response, and candida. She was a mess physically and emotionally, since she had lost three babies in a row. Once or twice a day she would look at herself with hatred. She felt deeply disconnected.

At this time, her allergies were so severe that she was always blowing her nose, she had itchy eyes that would swell shut, and her face would get puffy. This is the rest of her story in her own words:

When my allergies kicked up, my face was so chapped, I would carry around wads of Kleenex and a small face towel. But Dr. Brantley's program was so powerful, my allergies cleared up in no time. In the years that followed, I only had two allergic attacks, once when I decided to eat four Dodger dogs. The next day Dr. Brantley laughed, and it was good to know that the program worked. When you get off the program (eating junk and non-foods), your body tells you immediately that it's out of balance. When I cheated, I could almost feel the histamine starting to be produced again. All these years later, if I slip and eat bread, my allergies immediately come back. It's just not worth the temporary pleasure.

Dr. Brantley's system was not complicated and neither were his principles. He explained that live foods begat live tissues, and dead foods begat dead tissues. Eat food from the earth, he told me, and nothing from a jar, can, or package. Vegetable juices are essential, and I was told to go no more than four hours between meals.

The diet allowed no caffeine, no sugar, and no bread. I was to drink vegetable juices, not fruit juices, and let me tell you, never in a million years did I think I could drink something green. I just couldn't face it at first, so I started with carrot and orange juice, but it was way too sweet for me. I changed to celery and cucumber juice, and to this day I'm addicted to it. In fact, there is nothing like it first thing in the morning, fresh out of the juicer.

I needed to drink water all throughout the day, and lemon and water in the morning. Water was a critical part of the program, and it completely changed my eliminations. I took Dr. Brantley's enzymes and did liver/gallbladder flushes and all kinds of cleanses. But the real challenge for me was following the simple things he told me to do. It wasn't easy! Previously, food had controlled my thoughts, my moods, and there was a constant noise in my head. Food was a reward, it was a punishment, and always a friend. My body had betrayed me, I was angry, and I was on antidepressants, cutting myself out of every picture that was taken of me. I was obsessed about aging and plastic surgery and I couldn't even look in the mirror at my reflection without feeling disgusted. Most of all I felt dead inside, as if I were just going through the motions, disconnected with my body, sure that it had betrayed me.

Breaking the bond of tyranny with food results in freedom from all things. I can still remember how trapped I felt, how hard I worked, and how sad I was. I'd be driving home at midnight, catch sight of a Carl's Juniors, and I would pull in. I would eat that hamburger and fries, which made me feel better temporarily, but very soon I felt awful because I was eating the wrong foods. I was so addicted to fast food!

Then a shift occurred. Dr. Brantley told me that if I would take responsibility for what I put in my body, I would undoubtedly see a change. I was sick and tired of food controlling most of my thoughts, and I was looking forward to breaking these shackles once and for all. And so, on April 2, 1999, I cut out all junk foods and bad foods, cold turkey. I wanted to lose weight and be thin, healthy, and free. I wanted to own my power, to wear a tennis dress, and to tuck my shirt into my jeans. And I didn't want to be embarrassed every time I got invited to a pool party.

I remember before the program, I'd resigned myself to the fact that I was getting old, that I was over the hill, fat, unattractive, and flawed. But when I started to do the program, I got plugged back into my body. Take it from me, anyone can rediscover their spiritual, sexual, and emotional selves because it doesn't work to attach to the sadness, grief, and despair. It felt great to fall asleep at night knowing I was doing everything as healthily as I could for my own body. Things were definitely changing.

The first change I noticed was in my elimination. After years of chronic cramps, constipation, and diarrhea, I started taking

Dr. Brantley's total body detox. My jeans became looser, and the more weight I lost, the better I felt and the more confidence I had in myself. My motivation and drive were stronger than ever, and my desire to get my elimination back in balance was foremost in my mind. I was confident that I was going to achieve optimal health, and that is exactly what happened.

As the pounds fell off, I knew it was not about weight loss but about health. Three months after I started the program, I walked into a clothing store, and for the first time in my life, I bought a petite-sized jacket. I was getting in tune with life and I loved walking the hills, drinking vegetable juice in the morning, and falling asleep at night, tired from the day, not from antidepressants. I loved the feeling of waking up with a bounce and hope— not feeling stiff, exhausted, and beaten up.

I know that part of the change came from the exercise that Dr. Brantley said I had to do. I started with light walking and tennis once a week. One month later, I was walking with a light run and I was still playing tennis. In another month, I was walking up hills, I began running, and then I started running up hills. Between running, tennis, and Pilates, the more I did, the more I wanted to do, and my energy increased. Dr. Brantley also told me to jump on the minitrampoline to break up trapped plasma proteins. But the main thing he stressed was that I had to do something physical every day, and if I did it in the morning, he promised it would kick-start my metabolism.

But here was my body's greatest accomplishment. In one year, my weight went from 186 down to 144, my waist went from $37\frac{1}{2}$ inches to 30 inches, my hips went from 47 inches to 39 inches, and I went from wearing a size 16 to a size 8! This time I was not on some crash diet. Rather I was eating to get healthy, and my body changed.

I remember Dr. Brantley coaxing me, "Claim it, Madeline. Own that power. I told you what to do, and you did it. You get as much out of the program as you put in. If you want to cheat 20 percent of the time, then you'll achieve 80 percent success. But if you do the program 100 percent, then the program gives you back 100 percent. There's no mystery to this program. People look at the outside of your body, where they can see the changes. But the changes within are too profound for words to describe!"

I look back to that time now, I remember how sad and angry I was back then, and I owe so much to Dr. Brantley. Through his program, he lifted my horrible guilt of losing those babies and he saw through my denial. He made me stop and take responsibility, encouraging me not to draw on the past, but to recognize all I had accomplished and to take a stand. He took me on a journey that I never knew was possible.

Once I stopped feeling like a victim to whom God had done something bad, and once I took responsibility for everything that went into my mouth, my whole world shifted. I stopped blaming other people or circumstances, I took responsibility for my own misery, and I realized that in some way, I was responsible for the outcome. I am the landlord of my body! The day I realized that, all blame went away and it was all about me and me. "It's so simple," Dr. Brantley said. "You don't need to do a million things. Just take responsibility for everything single thing that goes in your mouth."

Recently someone asked me, "Don't you miss ham sandwiches?"

"Well, sometimes I miss them," I said, "but I tell you what I don't miss—having tissues wadded up in my hands, or when I went to an event, hoping I wouldn't suddenly have a sneezing attack. I don't miss the dread of having someone's perfume kick me into a twelve-hour allergy spiral. I don't miss that at all. So if it means I have to give up a ham sandwich, that's okay by me."

Nothing feels as good as when you're eating the right things, drinking enough water, and taking care of yourself, because your body rewards you with an indescribable feeling. The best thing we can do for ourselves is to feed our body what it needs.

My medical doctor recently told me that my estrogen levels had dropped, that I needed to watch my blood sugar levels, and it didn't faze me a bit. Armed with everything that I learned from Dr. Brantley, I knew exactly what to do. I instantly increased my water intake, cut out my fruit in the morning, and got back on my exercise program. I thought, *Thank you very much for reminding me that there are no shortcuts. You need to keep doing the work, and there you have it. All I need to do is remove the cause. There are no mysteries here anymore.*

There is nothing left for me to say. I only hope that you commit yourself to this program 100 percent, as Madeline did.

Balance your life: *You are the cure!*

CHAPTER 18

The Antiaging Cure

What's Aging You?

Do you ever wonder what is really aging you? Imbalances from poor eating habits, pharamceutical drugs, and environmental poisons could cause toxins to build up, causing rapid destruction and deterioration at the cellular level. At the same time, our bodies are sustaining free-radical damage every moment of the day, aging our tissues, glands, organs, and skin.

As our cells use oxygen to make energy, they produce free radicals as a result of the body's everyday functions such as digestion, metabolism, and circulation. Free radicals also are produced from air pollutions, pesticides, cigarette smoke, and common household cleansers, to name just a few. These unstable molecules bounce all around the body, like hot BBs, and whatever they hit, they damage. If we are looking at wrinkled skin with liver spots, those are only the outward manifestations of free-radical damage. Behind the scenes, our organs, glands, tissues, and muscles are suffering damage as well, and this free-radical damage can lead to cancer and other degenerative diseases.

At first it was commonly believed that free radicals damaged the DNA of the cell. Then in 1978, Imre Nagy, M.D., a Hungarian scientist, analyzed cells taken from people who were a hundred years old to find that their cells still could reproduce and their cell DNA was not damaged. Through years of research, Dr. Nagy concluded in his thesis about the membrane hypothesis of aging that free radicals did most of their damage to the outer layer of the cell, not the DNA. Once the cell membrane was damaged, it started to lose its ability to let nutrients in and waste out. As the waste and salts such as potassium began to build up, taking up precious room inside the cell, the water inside the cell was forced out and the cell became dehydrated.

With all this daily damage to our cells going on, they survive because the body has built its own defense system, antioxidants, which help fight free radicals. Antioxidants give the free radical the electron or electrons it needs by latching onto it. When these join together, the free radical is satisfied and no longer tries to latch onto any other parts of the cells.

If we add insult to injury and feed ourselves worthless nonfoods, our personal storehouses of antioxidants get used up and we end up aging prematurely. That is why a diet rich in organic raw fruits and vegetables full of antioxidants is essential to protect us from this constant barrage. Also, rest and relaxation are absolutely necessary if the body is to repair what has been damaged by the process of life.

If we want to look younger and feel younger, we need to get ourselves in bed at a decent hour. If we are stressed, it shows on our skin, and proper hydration is vitally important. A friend of mine can look like she has aged ten years from one day to the next if she is stressed and not hydrated. You bet she drinks her pure water!

Another reason for aging is a reduction of the amount of human growth hormone (HGH) our body produces, starting in our twenties. Please visit my Web site for additional information about HGH, antiaging formulas, and skin products.

Tony's Story

Whether or not you care about wrinkles, everyone cares about energy. When you're young, it felt like you could go on forever, working for eight to ten hours, coming home and partying all night, and repeating this over and over again. But not many of us can keep that up after a certain age. We just get too pooped out. We work, come home, and flop on the couch, barely able to walk to the kitchen and make dinner—and the energy drain seems only to worsen with each birthday. For my client Tony, this situation was compromising his career, his relationships, and his state of mind. He was completely and utterly exhausted, and he didn't have the faintest idea why.

Tony's wife had come to see me some months earlier, and he was so impressed with the changes he saw in his wife, he wanted to see me, too. He arrived for his first appointment in 1994, totally lethargic, standing five foot eleven and weighing 196 pounds. "When I get in the shower in the morning," he said, "I'm so tired, I'm almost in tears from the sheer exhaustion. It's been going on for two to three years now."

He explained that somehow he had adjusted by performing well at work. At home, he had no interest and no energy: "I just can't get enthusiastic about anything."

Tony was fifty-eight years old, and he had no idea how his diet was affecting his health. He'd go to work and eat whatever the cafeteria served for lunch, which was bacon, eggs, sandwiches, or something else equally junky. He ate a lot of sugar, and I was stunned when he told me that he drank fifteen to twenty cups of coffee a day. He had given up smoking in 1974, but before that, he had smoked about ten cigarettes a day for about 23 years.

He had other symptoms, too, but Tony was in such denial, he was not aware that he had shortness of breath until I pointed it out during his first appointment. He'd walked up the stairs and was breathing very hard when he entered my office, but he paid no attention because he was so accustomed to having these symptoms.

After the first appointment, I gave Tony a nutritional program and he went on it strictly, even though he had never done anything like that in his life. That was in November, and his second daughter was getting married in April. He wanted to feel better by April, and when he started on my dietary and herbal suggestions, he noticed an energy difference in one week. Every week thereafter, he felt better and better until his fatigue disappeared completely.

Previously he had been out of touch with how his body reacted to things, and it usually took him twice as long to get results. But when he took my herbal formulas, he got an immediate feeling of well-being in his body. "It made me want to double the dose," he said, "but I never did!

I just wanted to keep taking the stuff forever, because they made me feel so great. Even to this day, I love Timothy's herbal formulas and won't be without them."

He was improving his health in every area of his body, and by April, Tony had gone from 196 pounds to 163 pounds, just in time to walk his daughter down the aisle. And all he did was eat properly and eliminate coffee and sugar. He was not trying to lose weight, but he was happy that it happened anyway.

By the time his daughter's wedding arrived, he was feeling so good, he was coping easily with all kinds of stress, and he never knew that he could feel that good. It's been twelve years now and he says, "Sometimes I wonder if I'd even be here without Timothy, because I was declining much too quickly."

It has been my privilege to work with Tony and his wife, Frances, who say they couldn't feel better. Tony told me that he feels better today than when he was a kid. He says, "I marvel at how splendid it feels to be so committed to doing the work." Our body definitely rewards us. It's so simple.

A Final Word:
Health Is Your Divine Birthright

Imagine living in a healthy and vibrant body, feeling great every day of your life. What if I told you this is not a fantasy? The truth is that you already live in a body designed for balance and optimal health. In fact, health is your divine birthright, the condition that our Creator had in mind for each one of us.

Your body knows only one thing for sure—how to balance, heal and restore itself—if you allow it to do so. Balance equals optimal health, and the body was designed to constantly return to balance and health because diseases cannot live in a healthy body. All you have to do is follow Creation's road map to balance, outlined here in the pages of this book.

I gave you the keys in the previous pages and now it's up to you to pick it up and claim your birthright by creating a healthy inner environment. You hold the key to health, so let's go back over the basics:

- Follow the rules and laws of Creation—the only real authority.
- Live according to Creation and remember that prevention is the key.

- Always keep the idea of balance in the forefront of your mind.

- Understand what you have learned and why it works.

- Ask questions when you don't understand, and don't stop until you get an answer.

- Take responsibility for your actions and what you put in your mouth.

- Don't wait until you're in trouble to take action.

- You are your best health insurance policy.

A long, fulfilling life of optimal health is possible for everyone, because with your support, the body can heal itself of anything! I am a living, breathing testimony to that, since the medical doctors told me that I would have to live with my condition for the rest of my life. I would not accept that, and neither should you. When it becomes clear to you that the very people you turn to for health problems do not understand the laws of Creation, the only real healer, it's time to look elsewhere.

The bottom line is that only what comes from Creation is correct for the human body. This truth always was and always will be. My clients, over two decades, agree that Creation saved their lives, even after the traditional medical community gave them no hope. Thank God the powers that be were wrong and Creation was right. It has always been right, and I have been fortunate to rediscover the only real authority over the health of human beings—Creation itself.

Just look at the brilliance with which we were designed, created to live in optimal health utilizing the foods that come from the earth and the sea. Nothing made by man ever has touched or ever will touch the perfection of what is made by Creation—the only true and correct building blocks that should enter the human body. These magical elements are correct for us as food, drink, and medicine. We need nothing else. Do you think you're worth it? Do you love and respect yourself enough to be your own best health authority and to make the choices that will benefit your mind, body, and spirit?

To reiterate, your best health insurance policy is all about the choices you make concerning what you put inside your body. The dividends you get back will either be sickness and disease or balance and optimal health. It really is up to you. Now that you know what to do and how to do it, why not make the choices that will bring you great health and satisfaction as you live among the magnificence of what God created for us? Never forget that no matter how sick you are or what anyone has to say about it, *you* can heal *you*.

Balance your life. *You are the cure.*

AUTHOR'S PRODUCTS

Brantley Wellness Formulas

In a world where it is questionable to trust the myriad of herbal, nutritional, and homeopathic products available, where do you turn for advice? How do you choose what is correct for you and can help reverse your health challenges? Let's go back to our roots—to the earth, to the healing herbs and foods that Creation has provided. There you will find your answers. I looked there when I was a teenager, and I can honestly say that nature has never let me down. My formulas are based on the statement of Hippocrates "Let your food be your medicine and your medicine be your food."

I am thrilled to offer you many of the same herbal/food combinations that I have personally researched and crafted over the years for my clients, family, and friends. Creation labored to offer us these natural healing substances, and my particular gifts led me to create different ways of putting those herbs together.

Working with healing herbs and food is my passion, and I have lived a life knee-deep in herbal formulas for more than twenty years. I formulated these remedies for many of my clients who were literally dying, and I was their only hope. I called on every scrap of knowledge and instinct I possessed to make my formulas so powerful that they could kick-start the weakest and most debilitated systems. These formulas were not conjured on paper or copied from a book. I tested them in my clinic on critically ill clients over the past twenty years, and they have saved thousands of lives because they are so strong.

As an herbalist, a naturopath and a Ph.D., I don't mess around. Great results are my only option. With my priority testing method, I make certain, beyond a shadow of a doubt, that the individual herbs in my formulas not only complement one another energetically, but also are the most powerful combination of herbs on the planet.

My life's mission is to source the highest-quality herbs and use them in my herbal formulas. All you need to do is cleanse and feed your body with the most powerful medicinal elements known to man, provided by Creation, and then let your body do the healing. Remember: *You are the cure.*

The Brantley Essentials Product Line

The following three formulas make up the Brantley Essentials Quick Start Program. Sadly, if we had relied less on quick-fix drugs and instead directed its focus to prevention through following Creation's laws, disease statistics would not be sky-high. Prevention is the key! Don't wait for a scary diagnosis to elicit change. All my clients have used my herbal formulas not only to encourage their bodies to heal, but also to keep themselves vibrantly healthy. Take my herbal formulas to prevent serious illness and premature aging. The name of the game is: nutrition in + waste out = supercharged organs and cells.

Active Enzymes *Plus*: The Fountain of Youth

If you still eat cooked food or you have lost some of your digestive capability, consider taking digestive enzymes with each meal. When you cook your food, many important enzymes that would normally help break down food are destroyed. As we eat more and more cooked food over time, our enzyme reserves may get depleted and our health and our immune systems may be compromised. The Brantley Active Enzymes *Plus* Formula supports the digestive process by helping to digest and break down fat, protein, and carbohydrates, supplying a rich supply of enzymes for your body. The Brantley Active Enzymes *Plus* Formula provides support for your overburdened liver, pancreas, and gallbladder, which have been working overtime to try to digest cooked and processed food. Because many of us have never cleansed our livers and gallbladders, they may be clogged and may not be working to capacity. If you have indigestion, gas, bloating, constipation, or acid reflux, this may be an indication that your digestive process is compromised. Taking the Brantley Digestive Enzyme Formula at every meal insures your ability to fully break down food and utilize the nutrients inherent in the food source.

Brantley Live Food Buffet

As streams of sick and dying clients flooded through my clinic, each was in a state of cellular starvation. Their bodies were failing because their cells, organs, tissues, blood, and brain were not being fed properly. Eating a few fruits a day and some vegetables at dinner was simply not enough. Behind the scenes, their body were struggling. Because they were severely malnourished, they were aging too quickly; their tissues and cells were dying; they were getting eaten up by free radicals, toxins, opportunistic parasites, bacteria, viruses, and fungi; and their immune and elimination systems couldn't keep up.

We can't afford to go one day without proper nutrition. Every day we do, we take one step backward toward exhaustion and disease. I created my Live Food Buffet powder with this in mind. I used the highest quality raw foods, unaltered and untouched, from the land and the sea. Live Food Buffet is literally a smorgasbord of nutrients that can feed your trillions of cells, balance your pH and body fluids, and give you enough antioxidant activity to win the battle and neutralize free radicals, which cause tissue damage, cell death, and premature aging. Live Food Buffet has enough raw and wholesome goodness to feed your body on a deep cellular level. Daily, it provides all the vitamins, macro- and microminerals, amino acids, essential fatty acids, raw fats, and enzymes in a form that is easily assimilated. Live Food Buffet is so alive and nutritious that over continued use it has the capacity to replenish years of nutritional loss. Listen to your body's many cries for nourishment. Add Live Food Buffet to my shake recipes in chapter 14 or visit my Web site at www.Brantleycure.com for additional recipes suggestions.

Brantley Cell Core

Our bodies are vulnerable to outside invaders when our systems are overloaded with toxins, stress, and junk foods. As a result, our intestines, liver and gallbladder, kidneys, and lymphatic system struggle to detoxify, and our white blood cells must embark on search-and-destroy missions to get rid of harmful undigested putrefied foods, bacteria, viruses, and fungi. Our immune defenses are continually trying to protect our cells from succumbing to infections or destruction. Many times, our overburdened immune system cannot keep up with such unreasonable demands. Our blood becomes jam-packed with recirculating toxins, and our health goes down the tubes. Our glands get swollen, we catch every flu or virus that comes our way, our energy drops, and/or our diagnoses become much more serious. To support our tired immune system and to dramatically increase our energy and feeling of well-being, I formulated Cell Core, which boosts the immune system and is a powerful blood cleanser, purifier, and detoxifier. It cleanses the lymph system and keeps the blood and tissues oxygenated. Keeping the body oxygenated, especially at the cellular level, can be an important factor in the prevention of cancer and other diseases. As this product encourages your body to eliminate waste, it helps balance the bodily fluids and normalize your pH. I used this formula with Kathy, Sonya, Howie, and other clients who had cancer, and I continue to use it in my clinic today. In my opinion, this formula was crucial in the reversal of cancer in the case studies cited in this book and should be taken regularly as a preventive measure to ensure optimal health and vitality.

Brantley Rescue Me

Let's face it—no one is perfect. No matter how much you commit yourself to a healthy and balanced diet, from time to time you are going to slip and fall. When that beer and hot dog are staring you in the face at the ball game, or that piece of chocolate mud pie is calling your name, there is no way that you are going to resist 100 percent of the time. And just think of what happens during the holidays: Halloween, Thanksgiving, Christmas, Hanukkah, and New Year. We all ingest enough sugar, white flour, and alcohol to devastate our immune defenses. And what goes on inside your body as you swallow this deluge of junk? It deoxygenates and acidifies your system, which can allow the development of colds, flu, cancer, and other diseases. Also, whatever nonfood is not digested ends up sticking to the walls of your intestines like toxic glue, clogging your intestinal tract, eventually leading to a plethora of health problems. To help avoid these problems, take Rescue Me. This two-product combo forms a protective shield that stops and washes away toxic residue, keeping it from causing not only short-term but long-term damage. Active Enzymes *Plus* can protect your organs, glands, and tissues from damage by breaking down harmful bits of junk food and junk drink. Total Body Detox washes away toxic debris and detoxifies your intestines, liver and gallbladder, kidneys, bladder, pancreas, adrenals, and blood. It cleans so deeply, that it can pull toxins out of your entire body, while most herbal cleansers only detoxify the large intestines. Rescue Me never gives junk food a chance to pollute your system. Instead of feeling nauseous, bloated, and headachy after eating junk, you can use Rescue Me to neutralize and wash away toxins before they have a chance to make you miserable. Take Rescue Me at night before bed, and you can feel great in the morning. Rescue Me also ensures that you will have a deep-cleansing elimination. Although I am not advocating falling off the healthy food wagon, I am realistic. When you eat something questionable, Rescue Me can protect you from damage.

The Brantley Essentials Quick Start Program is available on my Web site at www.Brantleycure.com.

The Brantley 7-Day Intestinal Detox Program

I have spent years in the pursuit of the best herbal combinations to cleanse the intestinal tract. After trying almost everything out there (often ripping up my insides with harsh herbal cleansers), I formulated an unbeatable combination of formulas. This 7-Day Intestinal Detox program is suggested for anyone who has ever, in their lifetime eaten at a fast-food restaurant or enjoyed pizza, sodas, alcohol, or a myriad of desserts and ice cream. If your eating habits have not been perfect, then you should detoxify your intestines. Death starts in your colon! One in every 2.5 people will die of some form of cancer, and the problem can start with intestinal toxicity. The following three formulas will help you start the process of cleaning out the toxic waste dump that may exist inside of you.

Brantley The Eliminator

Almost everyone has been carrying around an astronomical amount of toxins and undigested waste material in their small and large intestines. After surgery, doctors have been shocked to find as much as fifty pounds or more of excess waste crammed into those forgiving tubes! When you eat junk food and processed food, some of this indigestible, gross, and gluey substance deposits themselves on the intestinal walls, drying out and hardening your stool, making it difficult to move your bowels. When your bowels are plugged up and you are in constipation hell, this formula will open you up when you are in trouble. The Eliminator goes in and softens waste so these toxins can be eliminated. Whether you are starting an intestinal cleansing program or have just eaten the junkiest food imaginable, this product will move out the toxic debris painlessly, without abdominal cramping. Toxic waste and undigested food particles left stagnating in your intestinal tract lead to constipation, and constipation leads to ill health. Cleanse your way back to health. The Eliminator is also a natural, fast-acting herbal laxative. You can use it to alleviate constipation or use it regularly to help recorrect bowel movement regularity, without habit-forming side effects.

Brantley Smart Fiber Plus

After The Eliminator starts to soften toxins, the herbs in Smart Fiber Plus will then penetrate the walls of the intestines and start to peel away years of hardened mucoid plaque and undigested food particles. The cleansing action of these herbs can also expose pockets of parasites that may have been eating away at your intestinal tissue. Bloating and swelling of the midsection is a result of hardened mucoid plaque getting stuck to certain parts of the intestines. This in turn can cause blockages, narrowing the passageways through the intestines. Your bowel movements can become hard and thin. The longer this material is stuck, the more it dries out your feces, making bowel movements uncomfortable and unsatisfying. That is why the action of this formula is so important. Smart Fiber Plus acts like a broom, softening and sweeping away debris, dramatically increasing the size of your bowel movements. The Eliminator and Smart Fiber Plus are perfect synergistic partners, deeply cleansing the colon without cramping or bloating.

Brantley Total Body Detox

Now that you have started to soften and sweep away the toxic waste, the Total Body Detox comes in to protect and simultaneously detoxify your body. It is so efficient, it can detoxify your small and large intestines, liver and gallbladder, kidneys, bladder, pancreas, adrenals, and blood. To make it more effective, I added herbs to nourish all of the organs mentioned above as you cleanse. This formula also softens years of hardened material and toxins that are clogging your body and ushers them out. Taking this formula regularly is like hiring a cleaning crew. You need to take the trash out on a regular basis, and the Brantley Total Body Detox is an excellent means to inside cleanliness.

The Brantley 21-Day Parasite Detox Program

Brantley Parasites No More

If you have been impacted for years and are in need of a deeper cleanse, combine Parasites No More with the three formulas described above, protecting your body from the toxic effects of a parasite infestation. If your internal environment is in a constant state of garbage overflow, it is the perfect time for all kinds of unwanted parasites to proliferate. These creatures feed off human flesh, living off undigested food particles and unfriendly bacteria in the gut. They take up residence not only in your small and large intestines, but in other parts of your body as well. As you eat, parasites gobble up the nutrition that was intended for your body, not theirs! Parasites can steal approximately 80 to 90 percent of our nutrition and energy. If you suffer from extreme fatigue, it is quite possible that parasites are part of your problem. Intestines packed with sludge provide a perfect breeding ground where parasites can thrive for years. Parasite infestation is very prevalent, and you don't have to travel to distant lands for these parasites to flourish. Symptoms such as gas, bloating, anal itching, skin rashes, diarrhea, or abdominal discomfort could be signs that it is time to kill the parasites. I formulated Parasites No More for myself and my clients because I found the other herbal formulas to be ineffective. Critters of all kinds have no chance of surviving this strong and powerful parasite cleanser.

All the Brantley Intestinal Detox programs and individual formulas are available on my Web site at www.Brantleycure.com.

The Brantley 7-Day Liver/Gallbladder Detox

Brantley Liver Detox

No one would think of going too long without cleaning the oil filter in the car, but most of us never think about cleansing our liver. Your liver is the hardest-working filtering organ in our body. After a lifetime of improper eating, an unbalanced lifestyle, and junk-food binges, your liver gets dirty and clogged. When it does, you feel lousy and toxic. In fact, every critically ill client I have ever worked with had a liver that was overflowing with toxins. Day in and day out, the liver is our body's first defense. It filters out pesticides, chemicals of any kind, food additives and preservatives, prescription medications, over-the-counter drugs, alcohol, recreational drugs, artificial sweeteners, air pollutants, car exhaust, harmful fumes from carpets and paint, molds, dead parasites, bacteria, viruses, fungi, cleaning products, and allergens, to name just a few. The liver is also vital for hormone metabolism and digestion. If your liver was not able to perform this filtering function for even one day, your body would soon go into a state of toxic shock and you would die. Your liver is your protective shield that saves you from being poisoned by our toxic atmosphere and inferior food chain. If your liver is sick and tired, you are sick and tired. There is no doubt in my mind that you must cleanse your liver to achieve great health. If you have ever suffered from headaches, nausea, body aches, or obesity; if you have been diagnosed with a serious illness; or if you drink alcohol or take prescription or over-the-counter drugs, you need a liver cleanse. The Brantley Liver Detox formula has effectively cleansed thousands of people's livers over the years, with glorious results.

Brantley Gallstones No More

If you are cleansing your liver, you can't forget your gallbladder—they work as a team. The gallbladder stores bile coming from the liver. Bile has many functions. It contains neutralized poisons from the filtering action of the liver, and it stimulates digestion and emulsifies fats. If your gallbladder is clogged with toxins or hardened cholesterol molecules, neither organ can perform its functions and your digestion is greatly compromised. Within this congestion, gallstones form and get trapped, causing pain and nausea. That is why I created Gallstones No More. Add this formula to the daily drink discussed on page 180 to slowly soften, emulsify, and eliminate stones and years of accumulated hardenings in the gallbladder. If you have been diagnosed with gallstones or you experience symptoms such as frequent belching, gas, bloating, pain under your ribs on the right side, nausea, or intolerance of greasy foods, Gallstones No More works in conjunction with the Brantley Liver Detox formula. Even without these symptoms, there is a strong possibility that your liver and gallbladder are clogged and compromised from the immense amount of processed foods, toxic fumes, pesticides, food additives, dyes, preservatives, and prescription meds to which we have all been exposed. If this congestion remains, the ability of the gallbladder to participate in digestion and break down fats will be greatly compromised, leading to weight gain and an extended midsection. By using the Brantley Gallstones No More formula, you will help your body dissolve the stones that are trapped in the middle of this stagnated waste.

The Brantley 7-Day Liver/Gallbladder Detox program and individual formulas are extremely efficient at clearing out the debris in both the liver and the gallbladder. They are available on my Web site at www.Brantleycure.com.

The Brantley 7 Day Kidney/Bladder Detox Program

Brantley Kidney/Bladder Detox

Many times your kidneys and/or bladder may be filled with toxins, infection, or inflammation without your ever experiencing symptoms. The kidney's job is to filter your blood. First, the kidneys return clean blood back to the body, and then make urine to wash the waste out of the body. They also regulate the electrolyes and the pH balance of the blood. But if any filtering or elimination organ such as the kidneys can't keep up with the flushing process they will eventually become hardened with debris. When that happens, you can suffer from backaches, body aches, constant kidney and bladder infections, and edema. This is why it is critical to your health to keep these organs in perfect running order. Kidney/Bladder Detox cleanses, disinfects, and soothes, all at the same time. It can be taken for urinary tract infections (cystitis), including symptoms such as pain, burning, and frequent and/or urgent urination. If your urine is pungent or cloudy, if you have frequent lower backaches or frequent urination, or if you have taken prescription medications, I strongly recommend that you do this cleanse.

Brantley Kidney Stones No More

Once again, with a constant barrage of toxins circulating through your blood, it is no surprise that the kidneys and the bladder are subject to hardenings, calcification, and kidney stones. Along with the Brantley Kidney/Bladder Detox formula, use the Brantley Kidney Stones No More Formula to dissolve kidney stones and bladder calculus. We often live with these hardenings without any noticeable symptoms. If this is the case, your kidneys and bladder are not functioning properly and are not as efficient in filtering out poisons, excess protein by-products, and excess toxins that will be dangerous if not eliminated.

The Brantley 7-Day Kidney/Bladder Detox program is subtle but very effective in slowly dissolving and removing these obstructions. Before you go through the excruciating pain of trying to pass a kidney stone, cleanse these organs. It has proven to be extremely effective over the last twenty years in my clinical practice. The Brantley 7-Day Kidney/Bladder Detox program and individual formulas can be found on my Web site at www.Brantleycure.com.

How to Order Brantley Formulas

My products are not available in stores. To order, please go to my Web site at www.Brantleycure.com or call 1-800-560-CURE. On my Web site you will find the most comprehensive and current health and research resources available on the Internet, including:

1. Educational DVDs on cancer, obesity, heart disease, and blood sugar problems and detailed descriptions of intestinal, liver and

gallbladder, and kidney and bladder detox programs and proto-cols, to name a few

2. A comprehensive list of natural cancer treatments and clinics around the world

3. New Brantley Wellness Formulas

4. An updated list of my seminar tours and TV appearances

5. Information on where to purchase the healthiest waters

6. A list of natural doctors and healthcare professionals

7. A list of health food and/or raw food restaurants

All lists and services are constantly researched and updated.

BIBLIOGRAPHY

Alt, Carol. *Eating in the Raw*, New York: Clarkson Potter, 2004.

Baird, Lori, and Julie Rodwell, eds. *The Complete Book of Raw Food*. Long Island City, N.Y.: Hatherleigh Press, 2005.

Barefoot, Robert R., and Carl J. Reich, M.D. *The Calcium Factor*. Wickenburg, Ariz.: Bokar Consultants, 1992.

Batmanghelidj, F. *Your Body's Many Cries for Water*. Falls Church, Va.: Global Health Solutions, 1995.

Becker, Robert O., and Gary Selden. *The Body Electric*. New York: William Morrow, Quill, 1985.

Calbom, Cherie, and Maureen Keane. *Juicing for Life*. New York: Avery Books, 1992.

Emoto, Masaru. *The Hidden Messages in Water*. New York: Atria, 2005.

Goldberg, Burton. *Alternative Medicine: The Definitive Guide*. Berkeley, Calif.: Celestial Arts, 2002.

Gursche, Siegfried. *Healing with Herbal Juices*. Burnaby, B.C., Canada: Alive Publishing Group, 1993.

Howell, Edward. *Enzyme Nutrition*. New York: Avery, 1985.

Jensen, Bernard. *Tissue Cleansing through Bowel Management*. Escondido, Calif.: Bernard Jensen Enterprises, 1981.

Kulvinskas, Viktoras. *Survival into the 21st Century*. 21st Century Publications, 1975.

Mars, Brigitte. *Rawsome*. North Bergen, N.J.: Basic Health Publications, 2004.

Perricone, Nicholas. *The Wrinkle Cure: Unlock the Power of Cosmoceuticals for Supple, Youthful Skin.* New York: Rodale, 2000.

Rubin, Jordan S. *The Maker's Diet: The 40-Day Health Experiment That Will Change Your Life Forever*. Fayetteville, Ark.: Siloam Press, 2004.

Walker, N. W. *Become Younger*. Norwalk, Conn.: Norwalk Press, 1972.

——. *Fresh Vegetable and Fruit Juices*. Norwalk, Conn.: Norwalk Press, 1970.

——. *The Natural Way to Vibrant Health*. Ottawa, Ill.: Caroline House, 1976.

West, C. Samuel. *The Golden Seven Plus One: Conquer Disease with Eight Keys to Health, Beauty, and Peace*. Orem, Utah: Samuel, 1981.

INDEX

ABOUT THE AUTHOR

Dr. Timothy Brantley has been an independent researcher for more than twenty years, utilizing naturopathic principles. In his well-established practice in Santa Monica, California, he has been verifying his theories while working with thousands of clients over two decades. He received his Bachelor of Science degree from the University of Miami, two separate degrees in naturopathy from the Clayton School of Natural Healing and the International College of Naturopathy, as well as his Ph.D. from Pacific Western University. Dr. Brantley is a board-certified member of the American Naturopathic Medical Association.

With a natural affinity and talent for the healing arts, Dr. Brantley was drawn to medical alternatives and nutrition as a teenager, when his mother developed cancer. His unfortunate personal experience in watching her struggle and die deeply motivated his desire to learn to help people find ways to better support and maintain good health.

Born and raised in Miami, Dr. Brantley moved to Los Angeles to further his career in natural healing. Today his practice operates to capacity, and his expanding client list includes many celebrities. Dr. Brantley combines his communication skills with his extensive knowledge about health to fulfill his desire to help people attain optimal health.

Continually researching his clients' health challenges enables him to find exciting breakthroughs, which he now shares with the public. His mission is to empower people, showing them simple yet powerful solutions to their problems. Today he continues to formulate herbal and nutritional products, expanding his product line. He regularly appears on TV and radio shows, sharing his knowledge of and passion about health.